PHARMACOLOGY – RESEARCH, SAFETY TESTING AND REGULATION

ENVIRONMENTAL PHARMACOLOGY OF DICLOFENAC

PHARMACOLOGY – RESEARCH, SAFETY TESTING AND REGULATION

Additional books and e-books in this series can be found on Nova's website under the Series tab.

PHARMACOLOGY – RESEARCH, SAFETY TESTING AND REGULATION

ENVIRONMENTAL PHARMACOLOGY OF DICLOFENAC

EUGENIA YIANNAKOPOULOU
EDITOR

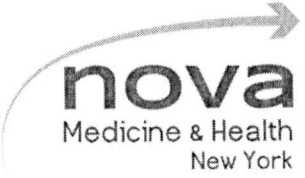

Copyright © 2020 by Nova Science Publishers, Inc.

All rights reserved. No part of this book may be reproduced, stored in a retrieval system or transmitted in any form or by any means: electronic, electrostatic, magnetic, tape, mechanical photocopying, recording or otherwise without the written permission of the Publisher.

We have partnered with Copyright Clearance Center to make it easy for you to obtain permissions to reuse content from this publication. Simply navigate to this publication's page on Nova's website and locate the "Get Permission" button below the title description. This button is linked directly to the title's permission page on copyright.com. Alternatively, you can visit copyright.com and search by title, ISBN, or ISSN.

For further questions about using the service on copyright.com, please contact:
Copyright Clearance Center
Phone: +1-(978) 750-8400   Fax: +1-(978) 750-4470   E-mail: info@copyright.com

NOTICE TO THE READER

The Publisher has taken reasonable care in the preparation of this book, but makes no expressed or implied warranty of any kind and assumes no responsibility for any errors or omissions. No liability is assumed for incidental or consequential damages in connection with or arising out of information contained in this book. The Publisher shall not be liable for any special, consequential, or exemplary damages resulting, in whole or in part, from the readers' use of, or reliance upon, this material. Any parts of this book based on government reports are so indicated and copyright is claimed for those parts to the extent applicable to compilations of such works.

Independent verification should be sought for any data, advice or recommendations contained in this book. In addition, no responsibility is assumed by the Publisher for any injury and/or damage to persons or property arising from any methods, products, instructions, ideas or otherwise contained in this publication.

This publication is designed to provide accurate and authoritative information with regard to the subject matter covered herein. It is sold with the clear understanding that the Publisher is not engaged in rendering legal or any other professional services. If legal or any other expert assistance is required, the services of a competent person should be sought. FROM A DECLARATION OF PARTICIPANTS JOINTLY ADOPTED BY A COMMITTEE OF THE AMERICAN BAR ASSOCIATION AND A COMMITTEE OF PUBLISHERS.

Additional color graphics may be available in the e-book version of this book.

Library of Congress Cataloging-in-Publication Data

ISBN: 978-1-53617-466-3

Published by Nova Science Publishers, Inc. † *New York*

CONTENTS

Preface		vii
Chapter 1	Environmental Pharmacovigilance *Syed Ziaur Rhman and Ahmad Zee Fahem*	1
Chapter 2	Environmental Pharmacology of Diclofenac with Special Reference to Vultures' Sensitivity *Syed Ziaur Rahman and Ahmad Zee Fahem*	23
Chapter 3	Environmental Toxicity of Diclofenac *Francis Orata*	41
Chapter 4	Source of Diclofenac in Drinking and Wastewater *Noshin Hashim, Aveen Alkhatib and Ajay K. Ray*	61
Chapter 5	From Environmental Pharmacology of Diclofenac to Human Pharmacology of Diclofenac: Implications for Human Health *Eugenia Yiannakopoulou*	87
Chapter 6	The Role of Oxidative Stress in the Environmental Toxicology of Diclofenac *Eugenia Yiannakopoulou*	105

Chapter 7	Methodological Issues in Environmental Pharmacology: The Paradigm of Diclofenac *Eugenia Yiannakopoulou*	**123**
Editor's Contact Information		**141**
Index		**143**

PREFACE

Nowadays, there is growing concern for the environmental risks of pharmaceuticals. Pharmaceuticals are present in the environment as a consequence of patient use, drug production and formulation, and improper disposal. Pharmaceuticals pose a risk for aquatic organisms as well as for terrestrial environment. Non-steroidal anti-inflammatory drug diclofenac is one of the most commonly prescribed medicines worldwide. Thus, there is growing concern for the potential environmental risks posed by diclofenac. Diclofenac has been included in the watch list of substances in EU that requires its environmental monitoring in the member states. Diclofenac has been shown to cause dramatic population declines (>99%) in Gyps vulture species in India and Pakistan, resulting in localised extinctions. Diclofenac has also been recognized as a threat for plants. Environmental toxicity of diclofenac in plants has implications for human health. Potential human exposure to diclofenac and diclofenac metabolites through dietary intake should be taken into account. Diclofenac as wells as other medications and personal care products may contaminate food produce via plant uptake, thus constituting a route for human exposure.

This book presents current knowledge on the environmental pharmacology of diclofenac, taking into account the potentially toxic effect of diclofenac in different eco-systems. In addition, using diclofenac as a paradigm, the book focuses on the discipline of eco-pharmacovigilance as well as on research methodology issues in the field of eco-pharmacovigilance.

All the chapters are well-written and structured and appropriately referenced. The most important feature of the book is that although the different chapters have been contributed by scientists with different fields of interest, the book can also be useful for medical doctors who are interested in the field of environmental pharmacology.

Environmental pharmacology is a multidisciplinary field of science. The book will be interesting for researchers with research interest in environmental pharmacology, i.e., pharmacologists, chemists, veterinary doctors, health policy makers, etc. The book will also be interesting for academic teachers, medical doctors, pharmacologists, pharmacists and medical students.

Chapter 1 - We are living in an environment that is polluted not only by heavy metals, pesticides, and emissions from gasoline engines, but also with pharmaceutical chemicals. Some drugs lead double lives! Once APIs in administered medications have completed their intended purposes, they can take on renewed lives in environment. These pharmaceuticals enter into environment through various routes causing harmful effects. Moreover, there is little concern and research to find adverse effects on environment, of particular drugs given at therapeutic doses. A number of regulatory bodies like FDA and European Union have set some cut-off limit for environmental concentration of drugs. In Clinical Trials, where many limitations like that of limited size, narrow population, narrow indications and short duration are observed, the authors also found evaluation of drugs on environment is practiced very minimally. The Risk Assessment procedure for new active pharmaceutical substances, their metabolites, and also excipients, is to be done. The issue of potential impact of pharmaceuticals on environmental, is emerging one, but not new. The US-FDA has regulated pharmaceuticals in environment since 1977 through environmental review process for NDA. In Europe, guidelines for ERAs have been available in draft since 1996, with most recent draft issued in June 2006 including recommendations for appropriate precautionary and safety measures to limit product's environmental impact. As a part of Good CT, studies on impact of particular drugs on environment should too be incorporated. The existing term 'Ecopharmacology' is too broad and not even defined in a clear manner. The term 'Pharmacoenvironmentology' seeks to deal with environmental impact of drugs given to humans and animals at therapeutic doses. Some concerns that need to be taken up under Pharmacoenvironmentology are that of drugs and their exact concentration in different components of environment including deterrent measures such as Ecofriendly techniques like bioremediation.

Chapter 2 - Pharmacovigilance is the study of adverse drug reactions in both human and veterinary medicine. It helps in providing safety data and adverse update of all drugs after marketing. Hence, in clinical trial, it is also called as post-marketing surveillance or phase IV. Impact of human and veterinary drugs on environment is another emerging problem. Recent withdrawal of Diclofenac use in veterinary medical sciences and many other such instances which have direct relation with environment heralded a new discipline which is described as 'Pharmacoenvironmentology.' Evaluation of potential environment risks posed by the medical product is thus needed. This impact should be assessed and, on a case by case basis, special arrangements to limit it should be envisaged. Rapidly dwindling population of vultures is one such example where in the last few decades there had been dramatic decline of vultures. The reason of this decline was detected after a large gap of time. These vultures were showing signs of renal failure. Later, it was found that the cause of the renal failure was diclofenac (an NSAID), derived from diclofenac treated animal carcasses. These vultures were scavengers of the environment, so their loss posed a massive damage to the ecosystem. Several strategies were devised to decrease the decline of vulture population. These strategies included banning of production and use of diclofenac in veterinary practice, replacement of diclofenac with other NSAIDs like meloxicam which did not pose similar threat to vultures. Captive vulture breeding program was also launched by several countries of South Asian region like India, Nepal and Pakistan to increase the population of vultures which were on the verge of extinction. Such proactive measures were used to counter the deleterious effect of diclofenac on the environment. Pharmaco-environmentology is new discipline to check the unintended damage to ecosystem, as the environmental threat posed by thousands of drugs is massive.

Chapter 3 - Diclofenac is a widely used medicine with a potent analgesic, anti-inflammatory, and antipyretic actions. As a result, it is approved for treatment of rheumatoid arthritis, osteoarthritis, ankylosing spondylitis, dysmenorrhea, ocular inflammation and actinic keratosis among other health conditions. However, diclofenac is banned for veterinary use in many countries due to its discovered toxicity to animals. Studies have demonstrated that diclofenac can elicit responses in aquatic organisms at relatively low concentrations. Diclofenac presence has been detected and quantified throughout the various environmental matrices. Among the matrices where quantifiable levels of diclofenac have been obtained are drinking water, groundwater, sediment and wastewater which is from wastewater treatment plants. Theses contaminants presence in environmental matrices acts as a source or discharge point of diclofenac pollution to non-target organisms. As a consequence, unmetabolized form of diclofenac may enter the food chain and thus increase the potential to course adverse health effects posed to human and other organisms. In Human, diclofenac consumption has been associated with side effects on the cardiovascular, gastrointestinal, hepatic and renal systems among others. To date, most control policy and measures on diclofenac are informed by its acute toxicity. However, chronic toxicity, synergistic or antagonistic effects of diclofenac molecule but its metabolites and products of their reaction with other environmental molecules present, should inform the future policy and directives. The aim of this chapter is to discuss the environmental toxicity of diclofenac. The chapter will also report the on the occurrence of diclofenac in various environmental matrices and evaluate the risk they pose to non-target organisms.

Chapter 4 - Water pollution has become an increasing problem due to population growth, industrialization, urbanization and shifting climate patterns and it's increasing the demand for potable water. Pharmaceutical compounds, personal care products and endocrine disrupting compounds make up a substantial portion of water pollution. One of the commonly and heavily used pharmaceutical active ingredients is Diclofenac (DCF). Both DCF and its byproducts were found to possess a bio-accumulative risk due to its steady input into recipient waters and found to have toxic effects on cell function of aquatic animals. The problem aggregated due to the unreliability of the available conventional water treatment methods. As a result, Advanced Oxidation Processes (AOPs) has emerged to address this issues. Photocatalysis is a unique growing AOP for water treatment process that can be an alternative and effective solution for DCF treatment found in water sources. In this chapter, the source of DCF and its toxic byproducts in water sources are explained. Treatment options for removal of DCF and other pharmaceutical contaminants are introduced. In addition, the mechanism of photocatalysis, in treating water pollution such as DCF is described.

Chapter 5 - Nowadays, there is growing concern on the environmental risks of pharmaceuticals. Pharmaceuticals are present in the environment as a consequence of patient use, drug production and formulation, and improper disposal. Pharmaceuticals pose a risk for aquatic organisms as well as for terrestrial environment. Non-steroidal anti-inflammatory drug diclofenac is one of the most commonly prescribed medicines worldwide. Thus, there is growing concern on the potential environmental risks posed by diclofenac. Diclofenac has been included in the watch list of substances in EU that requires its environmental monitoring in the member states. Diclofenac is known to harmfully affect several environmental species already at concentrations of ≤ 1 µg/l. Most importantly, the environmental impact of diclofenac has implications for human health. Diclofenac has been shown to cause dramatic population declines (>99%) in Gyps vulture species in India and Pakistan, resulting in localised extinctions. The vultures suffered from renal failure after feeding on dead cattle that had been treated with diclofenac. The population decline of vultures has huge ecological consequences, as vultures are natural scavengers that eliminate animal carcasses. Unfed animal carcasses pose a threat for human health. Diclofenac has also been recognized as a threat for plants. Environmental toxicity of diclofenac in plants has implications for human health. Potential human exposure to diclofenac and diclofenac metabolites through dietary intake should be taken into account. Diclofenac as well as other medications and personal care products may contaminate food produce via plant uptake, thus constituting a route for human exposure. For example, crops may take up pharmaceuticals and personal care products through their roots. The paradigm of diclofenac highlights the need for novel environmental policies. Current knowledge on the occurrence of diclofenac in the environment should be improved. Diclofenac might pose an environmental risk in freshwater as well as in treated wastewater. Potential harmful effects of diclofenac in the environment should be monitored. The discipline of environmental pharmacology should be included in the academic curriculum of medicine and the other health sciences. A multidisciplinary approach is needed for ensuring the environmental safety of diclofenac as well as of the other pharmaceuticals.

In: Environmental Pharmacology of Diclofenac ISBN: 978-1-53617-466-3
Editor: Eugenia Yiannakopoulou   © 2020 Nova Science Publishers, Inc.

Chapter 1

ENVIRONMENTAL PHARMACOVIGILANCE

Syed Ziaur Rhman and *Ahmad Zee Fahem*

Department of Pharmacology, Jawaharlal Nehru Medical College,
Aligarh Muslim University, Aligarh, India

ABSTRACT

We are living in an environment that is polluted not only by heavy metals, pesticides, and emissions from gasoline engines, but also with pharmaceutical chemicals. Some drugs lead double lives! Once APIs in administered medications have completed their intended purposes, they can take on renewed lives in environment. These pharmaceuticals enter into environment through various routes causing harmful effects. Moreover, there is little concern and research to find adverse effects on environment, of particular drugs given at therapeutic doses. A number of regulatory bodies like FDA and European Union have set some cut-off limit for environmental concentration of drugs. In Clinical Trials, where many limitations like that of limited size, narrow population, narrow indications and short duration are observed, we also found evaluation of drugs on environment is practiced very minimally. The Risk Assessment

---

* Corresponding Author's Email: rahmansz@yahoo.com.

procedure for new active pharmaceutical substances, their metabolites, and also excipients, is to be done. The issue of potential impact of pharmaceuticals on environmental, is emerging one, but not new. The US-FDA has regulated pharmaceuticals in environment since 1977 through environmental review process for NDA. In Europe, guidelines for ERAs have been available in draft since 1996, with most recent draft issued in June 2006 including recommendations for appropriate precautionary and safety measures to limit product's environmental impact. As a part of Good CT, studies on impact of particular drugs on environment should too be incorporated. The existing term 'Ecopharmacology' is too broad and not even defined in a clear manner. The term 'Pharmacoenvironmentology' seeks to deal with environmental impact of drugs given to humans and animals at therapeutic doses. Some concerns that need to be taken up under Pharmacoenvironmentology are that of drugs and their exact concentration in different components of environment including deterrent measures such as Ecofriendly techniques like bioremediation.

Keywords: pharmacovigilance, pharmacoenvironmentology, ecopharmacology

1. INTRODUCTION, CONCEPTS AND BACKGROUND

According to World Health Organization, Pharmacovigilance activities are done for monitoring, detection, assessment, understanding and prevention of any obnoxious adverse reactions to drugs at therapeutic concentration on animal and human beings. However, there is also a growing focus among scientists and environmentalists about impact of drugs on environment and surroundings. While the role of pharmacovigilance has long been focused on occurrence of adverse outcomes from intended use of pharmaceuticals in both humans and domestic animals, another responsibility has only more recently emerged — the need to also protect environment from unintentional contact with active ingredients in pharmaceuticals.

With growing technological advances, newer and more effective drugs are being manufactured and are used on an ever-growing scale for people with various medical conditions. With growing research in the field of ecology and environment, many adverse effects of these drugs on the environment have come to light. The first study that detected drugs in sewage took place in 1976 at Big Blue River sewage treatment plant in Kansas City (C Hignite, DL Azarnoff, 1977, 337). In the meantime, a number of findings related to rising levels of some drugs and their adverse effects on the flora and fauna has necessitated some action by regulatory agencies like FDA and European Union. Still, there is lack of substantial protocol for prospective monitoring of drug concentrations in environment and the evident adverse effects.

A number of studies measuring levels in surface water, groundwater and drinking water of some drugs given therapeutically to humans and animals including antibiotics, hormones, pain killers, tranquilizers, beta blockers and anticancers were found (Ettore Zuccato, et al., 2000, 1789; Sascha Pawlowski, et al., 2003, 57; M Cleuvers, 2004, 309; DB Huggett, et al., 2002, 229; FM Christensen, 1998, 212; KN Woodward, 2005, 149; ABA Boxall, et al., 2003, 287). Development of antibiotic resistance in pathogens in the environment owing to their exposure is the major concern. Some prominent examples of drugs causing harmful effects on environment are that of vultures' death after consuming carcasses of animals treated with Diclofenac sodium (GW Aherne, R Briggs, 1989, 735; SZ Rahman, RA Khan, 2006, 229), Ethinyl estradiol adversely affecting fish through its "feminization" of males (GW Aherne, R Briggs, 1989), antidepressant drugs like Fluoxetine (Prozac) triggering spawning in shellfish and traces of Cocaine detected in River Thames (SZ Rahman, RA Khan, 2006). A few drugs are so synthesized that they tend to persist in the environment even after their excretion. Clofibric acid in aquatic environment disturbing the local fauna is an example (for more examples, refer Table 1).

When a human or animal is given a drug orally, it may either be fully or poorly absorbed from gastrointestinal tract. Clearly, unabsorbed drug would pass into the environment along with faeces. When humans or animals are given drugs parenterally or orally, the drug may be metabolized to a greater or lesser extent and excreted into environment (including in exhaled air) as parent drug or metabolites, or as a mixture of both. It means that once they are excreted into environment, they enter food chains and concentrate as they move upward into larger predators (Klaus Kummerer, Giampaolo Velo, 2006, 371). Ecopharmacology (Ecosystem + Pharmacology) describes entry of chemicals or drugs into environment through any route and at any concentration disturbing the balance of ecology (ecosystem), as a consequence (to see examples, refer Table 1). If these drugs enter through living organisms via elimination subsequent to pharmacotherapy, it should be a specific domain of pharmacology and not of only environmental studies. This domain may be referred as *Pharmacoenvironmentology*. Apart from that, Ecopharmacology as a major term should be restricted to studies of "PPCPs" irrespective of doses and route of entry into environment. PPCPs comprise a very broad and diverse collection of groups of chemicals substances comprising all human and veterinary drugs (available by prescription or over-the-counter; including new genre of "biologics"), diagnostic agents, "nutraceuticals" (bioactive food supplements), and other consumer chemicals, such as fragrances, cosmetics and sun-screen agents, "excipients" (so-called "inert" ingredients), biopharmaceuticals, dyes, pesticides, and many others (CG Daughton and TA Ternes, 1999, 907). This broad collection of substances refers, in general, to any product consumed by individuals for personal health or cosmetic reasons. The term Pharmacoenvironmentology can be used for this specialty dealing specifically with pharmacological agents and their impact on the environment, after elimination from humans and animals as post-therapy. The existing term 'Ecopharmacology' is too broad and not even defined in a clear manner. The term 'Pharmacoenvironmentology' seeks to deal with the environmental impact of drugs given to humans and animals at therapeutic doses. Here, we provide an overview to this new dimension of pharmacovigilance, capturing its expanded role in environmental protection with the term "PharmacoEnvironmentology."

Table 1. Examples of Ecopharmacology and Pharmacoenvironmentology

Examples of Pharmacoenvironmentology	Examples of Ecopharmacology
Radioactive material being excreted by carcinoma patients	PPCPs
Humans pass medicines and supplements through their system	Pharmaceutical pollution
Vultures' death after consuming carcasses of animals treated with Diclofenac sodium	Minamata Disease; Fungicide induced mercury poisoning in Iraq
Estrogens cause feminization of male fish. Ethinyl estradiol adversely affecting fish through its "feminization" of males	Incinerators converting the biowaste into chemical waste and radioactive substances from incinerators
Antibiotics, hormones, pain killers, tranquilizers, beta blockers and anti-cancers given therapeutically and found in surface water. Antibiotic resistance in the acquatic environment.	Common Effluent Treatment Plants (CETPs)
Antidepressant drugs like Fluoxetine (Prozac) triggering spawning in shellfish. Prozac induces reproduction in shellfish	Accumulation and disposal of unwanted, leftover medications
Traces of Cocaine detected in River Thames even through sewage treatment plants	Occupational diseases
Aggressiveness induced in lobsters by antidepressants	Medicine in drinking water such as pesticides, chlorine, etc.
Drugs persist in the environment per se even after their excretion, e.g., Clofibric acid in aquatic environment	Unwanted drugs improperly disposed of in toilet or trash
Venlafaxine causes foot detachment of freshwater snail, changes memory in cuttlefish	Nuclear, Biological and Chemical (NBC) waste release in international waters

1.1 Pharmacoenvironmentology: Expanding the Scope of Pharmacovigilance

Environmental pharmacology is an emerging specialty of pharmacology. It is defined as effect of pharmaceuticals and house care products on environment and ecosystem. It involves the study of gene-environment interaction, drug-environment interaction and toxin-environment interaction, for which specific terminologies have been, used very appropriately, i.e., 'Ecogeneology', 'Ecopharmacology' and 'Ecotoxicology', respectively (Bosun Banjoko 2014).

'Ecopharmacology' as a broader term describes entry of both 'pharmaceutics and personal care products (PPCPs)' and 'industrial and chemical pollutants (IACPs)' into the environment by any route and at any concentration disturbing the balance of ecology (ecosystem), as a consequence. This impact of PPCPs and IACPs on environment cannot be a part of Pharmacovigilance activity by virtue of its definition (Rahman SZ, et. al 2007, 20).

Pharmacovigilance as defined by WHO is concerned with "therapeutic concentrations". Although, this definition is used in some countries but certainly not in the EU or US where it extends to misuse, abuse, overdose, etc., as well as to environmental effects (regardless of whether the dose was therapeutic or otherwise). The term 'Pharmacoenvironmentology' seeks to deal with the environmental impact of drugs given to humans and animals at therapeutic doses.

If the human or veterinary drugs enter environment causing obnoxious reactions subsequent to pharmacotherapy via elimination from living organism, then this concept was defined in a specific domain of Pharmacovigilance or more appropriately a part of Environmental Pharmacovigilance (Rahman SZ, 2006, 1). This specific domain was later on referred as PharmacoEnvironmentology in 2006 (Rahman SZ, 2006, 1). It was specifically dealt with pharmacological agents and their impact on the environment, after elimination from humans and animals as post-therapy.

Ironically, in response to the term, PharmacoEnvironmentology, many new mumbo jumbo words of expressions were later on suggested such as 'EcoPharmacovigilance' in 2007 (Velo GP, 2007, 919; Velo GP & Moretti U, 2010, 963), 'PharmEcovigilance' in 2008 (Daughton CG, 2008, 1069) and 'Ecopharmacostewardship' in 2010 (Taylor D, 2010, 105). The idea is same, the concept is same and even the subject is same, then why so many terminologies? In addition to this complexity, some authors even mixed-up

"PharmacoEnvironmentology" and "EcoPharmacology" as one concept, which further confuse the whole subject (Rahman SZ, 2015).

Some prominent examples of drugs differentiating EcoPharmacology and PharmacoEnvironmentology are given in (Table 1).

2. SOME SPECIFIC ISSUES IN PHARMACOENVIRONMENTOLOGY

1. *Modern Medicines in Drinking Water*

    A vast array of pharmaceuticals has been found in the drinking water supplies. To be sure, the concentrations of these pharmaceuticals are tiny, measured in quantities of parts per billion or trillion, far below the levels of a medical dose. Pharmaceuticals primarily enter wastewater treatment plants from two sources: 1) excretion by the human body; and 2) disposal of unused or expired medications down the toilet or drain. Hospitals and residences account for the majority of pharmaceuticals entering municipal wastewater treatment plants. The wastewater is treated before it is discharged into reservoirs, rivers or lakes. Then, some of the water is cleaned again at drinking water treatment plants and piped to consumers. But most treatments do not remove all drug residues (The Times of India, 2008).

    During the past decade, there has been growing concern about potentially adverse effects of pharmaceuticals released in the environment through treated wastewater. Because of the large number of pharmaceuticals and the high cost of testing, relatively little data is available on the presence of pharmaceutical products in natural water bodies. U.S. Geological Survey in 1999 and 2000 showed 80% of the samples were contaminated with one or more pharmaceuticals albeit at very low concentrations. These include prescription drugs such as acetaminophen, steroids, hormones, codeine, antibiotics, antimicrobials, antidepressants, over-the-counter medicines such as pain relievers, ibuprofen, cold/flu remedies, antiseptics; and veterinary medicines.

2. *Avermectins*

Diazinon, an organophosphorus, is highly toxic to earthworms and other terrestrial organisms as well as to bees (Larkin & Tjeerdema, 2000, 49). Concern has been expressed over the toxicity of avermectin endectocides used widely in large animal veterinary medicine. These include ivermectin, doramectin and moxidectin (a milbemycin). Avermectins and milbemycins are voided in faeces where they may continue to exert insecticidal effects. This might cause major environmental problems, not only due to potential effects on insect populations but also preventing biodegradation of animal dung (Doherty et al., 71). Avermectins have low toxicity to a wide range of terrestrial invertebrates but possess low phytotoxicity (Halley et al., 1993, 109). The results of a number of experimental studies have indicated adverse effects on dung fauna by avermectins such as ivermectin and abamectin, whereas levamisole, moxidectin, tiamulin, olaquindox, metronidazole and benzimidazole anthelmintics including fenbendazole and albendazole appear to have no significant adverse effects. The sustained bolus formulations of these compounds may offer greater risks than other modes of administration (Errouissi et al., 2001; 421). The dung from treated animals may be less attractive to dung fauna, of which reasons are unknown (Holter et al., 1993). Treatment with ivermectin might also contribute to reductions in phosphorus recycling but the evidence for this is limited (King, 1993, 261). The residues of ivermectin in dung pats are slow to decline (Sommer & Steffanson, 1993, 67). Other investigators have found no or little evidence for adverse effects of avermectins on dung fauna or on dung pat degradation (Barth et al., 1993, 215).

The issue of avermectins and their environmental effects remains a controversial area (Forbes, 1996, 567). The treatment of terrestrial animals for parasite control is seasonal, as is the breeding of dung fauna. The latter might be at less risk if the breeding season and the treatment seasons are separate, but there may be some degree of risk if coincidental, and the concentrations found may depend on a number of factors including the diets of the treated animals (Cook et al., 1996, 205), and not all cattle in a herd will necessarily be treated simultaneously (Roncalli, 1989, 173). Interestingly, the original environmental impact assessments of avermectins in US took into account patterns of use, toxicity, metabolic characteristics, predicted environmental concentrations and behaviour in the environment but no consideration was given to effects on dung pat degradation or dung fauna (Bloom & Matheson, 1993, 281). There are some parallels with the treatment of cattle using deltamethrin. Depending on the time they are treated, and their frequency of drug administration, the effects on insects in cattle dung were either negligible or significant. For example, concentrations in faeces after a therapeutic treatment were sufficient to kill adult dung beetles (Wardhaugh et al., 1998, 270). Nevertheless, attempts to control parasitic flies by treating with avermectins so that residues in dung exert a beneficial insecticidal effect have met with little or no success (Mahon & Wardhaugh, 2001, 120). On the other hand, cypermethrin and fluazuron had no adverse effects on survival and reproduction in dung beetles (Kryger et al., 2006, 597 & 2007, 380).

2.1 Pharmaceuticals as Environmental Pollutants

It is only natural that attention has been historically directed to maintain the health and safety of populations for which medications have been developed — humans as well as domestic animals. But many drugs lead double lives! Once the active pharmaceutical ingredients (APIs) in administered medications have completed their intended purposes, they can take on renewed lives in the environment. APIs from a large and diverse spectrum of pharmaceuticals can enter environment as trace contaminants, especially in water, at individual concentrations generally less than a part per billion (µg/L), but sometimes more. These trace residues may pose risk for aquatic life (Boxall et al. 2004, 1; Cleuvers 2003, 185; Jones et al. 2002, 5013; Kidd et al. 2007, 8897) and cause concern with regard to human exposure, such as with contaminated drinking water supplies or food sources (Daughton 2004, 2008).

The predominant route by which APIs gain entry to environment is via the discharge of raw and treated sewage contaminated with APIs. Residues of APIs that are administered parenterally or enterally are often excreted in feces and urine, and topically applied medications can be washed from skin during bathing. For most APIs, the fraction of unchanged, parent API transferred to the environment is attenuated as a result of metabolism or transformation within a sewage treatment facility (such as by microbial degradation). For some APIs, only a small percentage is ever transported to the environment. For others, this percentage can approach 100%. Biodegradation modifies chemical structure of active molecules, which in turn often results in a change in their physicochemical and pharmaceutical properties. Metabolism may lower activity or enhance water solubility; however, metabolism is frequently incomplete. Excretion rates range from 0 to 100%. It means that in many cases, a large portion of the drugs is not assimilated by the patient's body and excreted as feces, urine, vomit, etc. (K Kümmerer, 2004).

A secondary route of transfer of APIs to environment is from the purposeful, direct disposal of leftover or unwanted medications to sewers and trash. The relative significance of disposal with respect to excretion and bathing, however, is poorly understood and is debatable. These disposal of unwanted chemicals, getting rid of unused, unwanted, or expired medications can be a challenge. Pharmacies may send unused or expired medications back to the original manufacturer. Alternatively, they may employ a reverse distribution company to take care of manufacturer returns and incinerate those products that are non-returnable. However, little is available in the way of formal guidelines on drug disposal especially at the level of final end user-the patient. It is reported that approximately one third of the total volume of pharmaceuticals sold in Germany and 25% of that sold in Australia was disposed with household waste or down the drain (K Kümmerer, 2004).

2.2 Connections between Human and Ecological Health

The occurrence of API residues in environment makes obvious the connection that exists between the practice of medicine and the protection of environment. The two are intimately tied but little is recognized as such. The two share many commonalities and connections. Consider the processes of data collection, articulation of symptomology, epidemiology, diagnosis, mitigation/treatment, prognosis, determination of vulnerability, and pollution/disease prevention. Each of these plays a critical role in both healthcare and environmental protection — in the "ecology of health" and in the "health of ecology." Improvements in one can impart collateral, unanticipated improvements in the other (Daughton 2003a).

With a new, added focus on environmental protection, active programs in EcoPharmacology could play premier role in pollution reduction or pollution prevention with respect to release of APIs. By optimizing the consumption and usage of medications to achieve the best healthcare outcomes for consumers, nearly all of the sources of easily controlled, environmental release of APIs could be best managed. Although pharmacovigilance currently follows postmarket events for humans and animals, analogous events concerning the environment have been largely ignored. With no system in place to routinely detect and report abnormal effects in the environment, this gap would be filled by expanding the traditional domain of pharmacovigilance. Although, pharmacovigilance in the human medicines sector is a well-established discipline but it is much more youthful in the veterinary sector. However, the objectives of human and veterinary pharmacovigilance are identical, and those developed for human pharmacovigilance can be readily adapted for veterinary purposes:

ECOPHARMACOLOGY

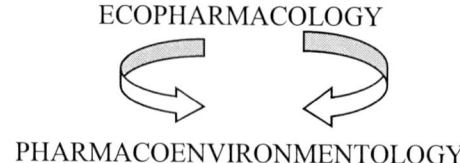

PHARMACOENVIRONMENTOLOGY

Figure 2. From echopharmacology to pharmacoevironmentology.

2.3 Life Cycle of Pharmaceuticals and Personal Care Products (PPCPs)

Although the concern on PPCPs in the environment is fairly recent, the problem cannot be considered as new. Pharmaceuticals have found their way into the environment for as long as they have been consumed. PPCPs may enter into the environment including drinking water. These substance xenobiotics in turn may enter into the human host and are eliminated from the human body through xenobiotic metabolism. Hepatic enzymes in liver primarily metabolize xenobiotics. The entry of these metabolites into the environment can occur through urine, feces, breath, and sweat. An understanding of xenobiotic metabolites is critical for the pharmaceutical industry because they are responsible for the breakdown of drugs. Most ingested drugs are excreted primarily through feces and urine in varying amounts of metabolized and unmetabolized forms. Metabolism may result in chemicals that are either more or less biologically active than the form in which they were consumed. While chemicals excreted as conjugates (combined with other chemicals in the body to make them water soluble) are usually biologically inactive, once in the environment, they can undergo hydrolysis, which can render them active, again (B Halling-Sorensen et al., 1998, 357). Sewage treatment facilities, depending on their technology and the chemical's structure, are not always effective in removing active chemical from wastewater. As a result, pharmaceuticals find their way into the aquatic environment, where they directly affect organisms and can be incorporated into food chains. Sources of input include direct dumping of excess or expired medication, as well as veterinary uses. With a growing population and an increased demand for medicine, the amount of PPCPs finding their way into the environment has been steadily increasing. (Anonymous, 2002b, 1).

It can be seen that there may be releases to the environment during the following stages: API synthesis, extraction and purification; commercial scale manufacture; animal/human clinical studies and use/disposal of unwanted pharmaceuticals.

3. SCOPE OF GUIDELINES ON ENVIRONMENTAL PHARMACOLOGY

3.1 Regulatory Measures

Though a number of regulatory bodies like FDA and European Union have set some cut-off limit for environmental concentration of drugs, no actual testing is conducted after a drug is marketed to see if the environmental concentration was estimated correctly.

When a new drug is proposed for market, FDA requires the manufacturer to conduct a risk assessment that estimates the concentrations in the environment. If the risk assessment concludes that the concentration will be < 1ppb, the drug is assumed to pose acceptable risks. FDA has never turned down a proposed new drug based on estimated environmental concentrations, and no actual testing is conducted after a drug is marketed to see if the environmental concentration was estimated correctly (Janet Raloff, 1998, 187). Apart from that there is little concern and research to find the adverse effects on environment, of particular drugs given at therapeutic doses. Even in clinical trials, where many limitations like that of limited size, narrow population, narrow indications and short duration are observed, we also found that evaluation of drugs on environment is practiced very minimally.

The European Union (EMEA Guidelines, 2006) has described a two-phased approach to evaluate Medicinal Products in environment. The environmental concentration of the medicinal product is calculated in

Phase I. Substances with a very high specific mode of action like hormones are directed to Phase II irrespectively of the result of exposure calculation. In the second phase, information on the physical, chemical and toxicological properties are obtained and assessed in relation to the environmental exposure of the medicinal product. Similarly, ERAs are also an integral part of the assessment process in the granting of marketing authorizations for veterinary medicinal products (KN Woodward, 2005, 149). According to John P. Sumpter (2007, 143), these recent EMEA guidelines covering the environmental risk assessment of human pharmaceuticals are a step in the right direction, but a more sophisticated approach, rather than a "one-fits-all" solution, is probably needed. As a part of a Good Clinical Trial, studies on impact of particular drugs on the environment should too be incorporated.

One topic that has been frequently discussed, but not sufficiently addressed is the environmentally safe disposal of pharmaceutical products. As a natural consequence of the supply chain process, from product development through patient usage, some products will inevitably be unused, damaged or will expire. Organizations such as WHO, World Bank, European Union and US-FDA have established some guidelines pertaining to this topic, but further action needs to be taken.

There is a dire need to provide countries struggling with product disposal with specific recommendations on how to properly dispose of products and to identify weaknesses within countries at all levels of the supply chain concerning unused, damaged or expired pharmaceutical products. For examples of situations occurring within specific countries or regions of where loopholes in the process exist and to what extent these problems have affected health care processes. This will allow us to document the scope of the problem and identify actions that need to eventually be taken on the national and international levels. Based on *WHO's Waste Management Guidelines* under the supervision of "Waste Management - WHO policy and activities", there is a need to further develop disposal recommendations for each of the medicines such as on the WHO List of Essential Medicines, 15th Edition.

3.2 Ecofriendly Techniques

Ecofriendly techniques such as bioremediation and phytoremediation may help in minimizing concentration of pharmaceutics, radionuclides, heavy metals and other pollutants especially organic compounds in acquatic environment. These techniques (bioventing, landfarming, bioreactor, composting, bioaugmentation, rhizofiltration and biostimulation) use microorganisms, fungi, green plants/transgenic plants or their enzymes to return the natural environment altered by contaminants to its original condition. These processes may also be employed to attack specific soil contaminants, such as degradation of chlorinated hydrocarbons by bacteria. An example of a more general approach is the cleanup of oil spills/grease spillage by the addition of nitrate and/or sulfate fertilisers to facilitate the decomposition of crude oil by indigenous or exogenous bacteria. There is a need of further 'screening of bio-molecules from microbial diversity collected from ecological niches'. Many as much as 200 bacteria including staphylococcus species and bacillus species have been identified from common effluent treatment plants (CETPs), which can break down some very tough molecules in wastewater. Wastewater, especially of industrial origin, contains not only harmful chemicals but such wastewater also supports the growth of many 'beneficial microorganisms', which might help to create or identify useful molecules for future cleanup of the industrial effluents. Some of these bacteria did not allow any other organism to grow around them, indicating their antibiotic properties. Characterization is needed before their molecules are extracted to be used in manufacturing drugs.

There should be some alternative avenues of disposing unused drugs. Like the use of incineration or chemical treatment plants to dispose of biomedical waste, there should be a solution for safe disposal of left over medicines. In biomedical waste management "polluter pays principle" should be followed. This means those who generate the waste must pay for its management. For example private nursing homes must pay municipal or BMW managing company for handling the BMW generated by individual facilities. For medicine waste, it should be "producer pays principle" which means that pharmaceutical companies must take back the expired medicines and ensure safe and scientific disposal. The pharmaceutical companies cannot just make the profits and get away. It is their responsibility to keep the world clean of the toxic effects of their produce. If the pharmaceutical industry is made accountable for the disposal of its unused produce, it can well recall all expired medicines and handle the same eco-friendly. The environment should not suffer because of disposal of expired medicines in garbage dumps. Medical and environmental ethics teach that if the medicines can do no good to people, these should do no harm also. Expired medicines should not "expire" the ecology. Hence the suggestion that "producer pays" because the "producer pollutes".

Conclusion

The pursuit of 'ideal' human pharmaceuticals is simultaneously driving improvement in its environmental profile that would lead to lower residues. Balancing the needs medicines and its potential environmental impact will continue to pose a challenge to society. WHO should frame guidelines such as "Guidelines for the Environmentally-Safe Disposal of Pharmaceutical Products" especially for Essential Medicines. Finally, the unknown is much bigger than the known but with the large uncertainties, it is best to limit release and exposure as much as practicable.

Pharmacovigilance pertains to the activities of adverse effects of drugs at therapeutic doses on animal and human beings. On the contrary, it is not possible to keep track of excreted metabolites of active or inactive ingredients as well as incompletely metabolised drugs into the environment. In this context, Pharmacoenvironmentology may be an extension of Pharmacovigilance dealing specifically with effects to the environment and ecology of drugs given in therapeutic concentrations. Pharmacologists having this particular expertise (pharmacoenvironmentologist) may be made a compulsory component of the team assessing different aspects of drug safety. We need to monitor the effects of drugs not only as a good medical practice, but also to safeguard our environment.

Wherever we live or travel, we impart unique chemical signatures on the environment in the form of minute residues of pharmaceuticals and personal care products that we excrete, wash from our bodies, or discard to sewerage or trash. While the contributions from each individual may be insignificant by themselves, the combined contributions from all individuals, as well as from medicated animals, reach measurable levels in surface and ground waters and on land receiving treated sewage (Daughton and Ruhoy, 2007, 1). Such is the importance of EcoPharmacology and PharmacoEnvironmentology. Since human and ecological health is intimately linked, efforts to improve one will inevitably lead to improvements in the other.

REFERENCES

Aherne GW, Briggs R. 1989. The relevance of the presence of certain synthetic steroids in the aquatic environment. *J Pharm Pharmacol* 41: 735–736.

Anonymous. 2002b. Pharmaceuticals in environment. Health Effects Review, *An official journal of Department of Environmental Health,* Boston University School of Public Health, 1-3.

Anonymous (2008). *Drugs found in drinking water*, The Times of India, March 10, 2008.

Barth D, Heinze-Mutz EM, Roncalli RA, Schlüter D & Gross SJ. 1993. The degradation of dung produced by cattle treated with an ivermectin slow-release bolus. *Veterinary Parasitology,* 48, 215-227.

Bloom RA & Matheson JC. 1993. Environmental assessment of avermectins by the US Food and Drug Administration. *Veterinary Parasitology,* 48, 281-294.

Bosun Banjoko. 2014. Environmental Pharmacology – An Overview (Chapter 5). *Pharmacology and Therapeutics,* InTech 2014.

Boxall ABA, Fogg LA, Blackwell PA, Kay P, Pemberton EJ, and Croxford A. 2004. Veterinary medicines in the environment. *Rev. Environ. Contam. Toxicol.* 180:1-91.

Boxall ABA, Kolpin DW, Sqrensen B, Tolls J. 2003. Are Veterinary Medicines Causing Environmental Risks? *Environmental Science & Technology* 287A-294A.

Christensen FM. 1998. Pharmaceuticals in the environment – a human risk? *Regul Toxicol Pharmacol* 28: 212-221.

Cleuvers M. 2003. Aquatic ecotoxicity of pharmaceuticals including the assessment of combination effects. *Toxicol. Lett.* 2003, 142(3):185-94.

Cleuvers M. 2004. Mixture toxicity of the anti-inflammatory drugs diclofenac, ibuprofen, naproxen and acetylsalicylic acid. *Ecotoxicol Environ Saf* 2004, 59: 309-315.

Cook DF, Dadour IR, Ali DN. 1996. Effect of diet on the excretion profile of ivermectin in cattle faeces. *International Journal for Parasitology,* 26, 291-295.

Daughton CG. 2003a. "Cradle-to-Cradle Stewardship of Drugs for Minimizing Their Environmental Disposition while Promoting Human Health. I. Rationale for and Avenues toward a Green Pharmacy," Environ. *Health Perspect.* 111:757-774.

Daughton CG. 2004. Groundwater Recharge and Chemical Contaminants: Challenges in Communicating the Connections and Collisions of Two Disparate Worlds. *Ground Water Monitor. Remed.* Daughton. 24(2): 127-138.

Daughton CG and Ternes TA. 1999. "Pharmaceuticals and Personal Care Products in the Environment: Agents of Subtle Change?" *Environ. Health Perspect.* 107(suppl 6), 907-938.

Daughton CG, Ruhoy IS. 2008. The afterlife of drugs and the role of PharmEcovigilance. *Drug Saf.* 31(12):1069-82.

Doherty WM, Stewart NP, Cobb RM & Keiran PJ. 1994. *In vitro comparison of the larvicidal activity of moxidectin and abamectin against Onthophagus gazella (F) (Coleoptra: Scarabaeidae) and Haematobia exigua De Meijere (Diptera: Muscidae). Journal of the Australian Entomological Society,* 33, 71-74.

Errouissi F, Alvinierie M, Galtier P, Kerbœf D & Lumaret JP. 2001. *The negative effects of the residues of ivermectin in cattle dung using a* sustained-release bolus on *Aphodius constans* (Duft.) *(Coleoptra: Aphodiidae)*. *Veterinary Research,* 32, 421-427.

Forbes A. (1996). Environmental assessments in veterinary parasitology: A balanced perspective. *International Journal of Parasitology,* 26, 567-569.

Halley BA, Van den Heuvel WJA & Wislocki PG. 1993. Environmental effects of the usage of avermectins in livestock. *Veterinary Parasitology,* 48, 109-125.

Halling-Sørensen B, Nielsen SN, Lanzky PF, Ingerslev F, Lüzhøft HCH, Jørgensen SE. 1998. Occurrence, fate and effects of pharmaceutical substances in the environment-A review. Chemo-sphere 36:357-393.

Hignite C, Azarnoff DL. 1977. Drugs and drug metabolites as environmental contaminants: chlorophenoxyisobutyrate and salicylic acid in sewage water effluent. *Life Sciences* 20: 337-341.

Holter P, Sommer C & Grønvold, J. 1993. Attractiveness of dung from ivermectin-treated cattle to Danish and afrotropical scarabaeid dung beetles. *Veterinary Parasitology,* 48, 159-169.

Huggett DB, Brooks BW, Peterson B, Foran CM, Schlenk D. 2002. Toxicity of Select Beta Adrenergic Receptor-Blocking Pharmaceuticals (B-Blockers) on Aquatic Organisms. *Archive of Environmental Contamination and Toxicology* 43 (2): 229-23.

Jones OA, Voulvoulis N, and Lester JN. 2002. Aquatic environmental assessment of the top 25 English prescription pharmaceuticals. *Water Res.* 36(20):5013-22.

Kidd KA, Blanchfield PJ, Mills KH, Palace VP, Evans RE, Lazorchak JM, and Flick RW. 2007. Collapse of a fish population after exposure to a synthetic estrogen. *Proc. Natl. Acad. Sci.* USA, 104(21): 8897–8901.

King KL. 1993. *The potential for avermectins to affect the nutrient economy of grazed pastures. Veterinary Parasitology,* 48, 261-271.

Kryger U, Deschodt C, Davis ALV & Scholtz CH. 2006. Effects of cattle treatment with a cypermethrin/cymiazol spray on survival and reproduction of the dung beetle species Euoniticellus intermedius (Coleoptra: Scarabaeidae). *Bulletin of Entomological Research,* 96, 597-603.

Kryger U, Deschodt C, Davis ALV & Scholtz CH. 2007. Effects of cattle treatment with a fluazuron pour-on on survival and reproduction of the dung beetle species Onthophagus gazelle (Fabricus). *Veterinary Pathology,* 143, 380-384.

Kümmerer K. 2004. Chapter 34, Conclusion in Klaus Kummerer (ed) *Pharmaceuticals in the Environment Sources, Fates, Effects and Risks,* Springer, New York, New York.

Kümmerer K, Velo G. 2006. Ecopharmacology: A New Topic of Importance in Pharmacovigilance. *Drug Safety* 29 (5): 371-373.

Larkin DJ. & Tjeerdema RS. 2000. Fate and effects of diazinon. *Reviews of Environmental Contamination and Toxicology,* 166, 49-82.

Naidoo V, Wolter K, Cromarty AD, Bartels P, Bekker L, McGaw L, et al. 2007. The pharmacokinetics of meloxicam in vultures. *PLoS ONE* 2:e686.

Oaks JL, Gilbert M, Virani MZ, Watson RT, Meteyer CU, Rideout BA et al. 2004. Diclofenac residues as the cause of vulture population decline in Pakistan. *Nature* 427: 630–3.

Pawlowski Sascha, Ternes Thomas, Bonerz Martin, et al. 2003. Combined in Situ and in Vitro Assessment of the Estrogenic Activity Sewage and Surface Water Samples. *Toxicological Sciences* 75: 57-65.

Prakash V. 1999. Status of vultures in Keoladeo National Park, Bharatpur, Rajasthan with special reference to population crash in Gyps species. *J Bombay Natural History Society* 96: 365-378.

Rahman SZ and Khan RA. 2006. Environmental pharmacology: A new discipline. *Indian J. Pharmacol.* 38:229-30.

Rahman SZ, Khan RA, Kumar V, Misbahuddin M. 2007. Pharmaco-environmentology – A Component of Pharmacovigilance, *BMC Environmental Health* 6:20 (http://www.ehjournal.net/content/6/1/20).

Raloff J. 1998. *Drugged Waters. Science News* 153 (12): 187-189.

Roncalli RA. 1989. Environmental aspects of use of ivermectin and abamectin in livestock: effects on cattle dung fauna. In *Ivermectin and Abamectin.* Ed Campbell, W.C. pp. 173-181. Springer-Verlag, London.

Ruhoy IS and Daughton CG. 2008. "Beyond the Medicine Cabinet: An Analysis of Where and Why Medications Accumulate," *Environ. Internat.* 34 (8): 1157-1169.

Sommer C & Steffansen B. 1993. Changes with time after treatment in the concentrations of ivermectin in fresh cow dung and in cow pats aged in the field. *Veterinary Parasitology*, 48, 67-73.

Sumpter John P. 2007. Environmental Effects of Human Pharmaceuticals. *Drug Information Journal* 41(2): 143-147.

Taylor D. 2010. *Ecopharmacostewardship: a pharmaceutical industry perspective.* In: Kümmerer K, Hempel M, editors. Green and sustainable pharmacy. Berlin/Heidelberg: Springer; 2010. pp. 105–126.

Velo G, Moretti U. 2010. *Ecopharmacovigilance for better health*. Drug Saf. 33(11):963–968.

Velo GP. 2007. Why EcoPharmacovigilance. *Drug Saf.* 30(10):919.

Wardhaugh KG, Longstaff BC & Lacey MJ. 1998. Effects of residues of deltamethrin in cattle faeces on the development and survival of three species of dung-beetle. *Australian Veterinary Journal*, 76, 273-280.

Woodward KN. 2005. Veterinary pharmacovigilance. Part 2. Veterinary pharmacovigilance in practice – the operation of a spontaneous reporting scheme in a European Union country – the UK, and schemes in other countries. *J Vet. Pharmaco Therap* 2005, 28: 149-170.

Woodward KN. 2005. Veterinary Pharmacovigilance. Part 3. Adverse effects of veterinary medicinal products in animals and on the environment. *J Vet Pharmacol Therap* 2005, 28: 171-184.

Zuccato Ettore, Calamari Davide, Natangelo Marco, Fanelli Roberto. 2000 Presence of therapeutic drugs in the environment. *The lancet* 355: 1789-1790.

In: Environmental Pharmacology of Diclofenac ISBN: 978-1-53617-466-3
Editor: Eugenia Yiannakopoulou   © 2020 Nova Science Publishers, Inc.

Chapter 2

ENVIRONMENTAL PHARMACOLOGY OF DICLOFENAC WITH SPECIAL REFERENCE TO VULTURES' SENSITIVITY

Syed Ziaur Rahman* and Ahmad Zee Fahem
Department of Pharmacology, Jawaharlal Nehru Medical College,
Aligarh Muslim University, Aligarh, India

ABSTRACT

Pharmacovigilance is the study of adverse drug reactions in both human and veterinary medicine. It helps in providing safety data and adverse update of all drugs after marketing. Hence, in clinical trial, it is also called as post-marketing surveillance or phase IV. Impact of human and veterinary drugs on environment is another emerging problem. Recent withdrawal of Diclofenac use in veterinary medical sciences and many other such instances which have direct relation with environment heralded a new discipline which is described as 'Pharmacoenvironmentology.' Evaluation of potential environment risks posed by the

---

* Corresponding Author's Email: rahmansz@yahoo.com.

medical product is thus needed. This impact should be assessed and, on a case by case basis, special arrangements to limit it should be envisaged. Rapidly dwindling population of vultures is one such example where in the last few decades there had been dramatic decline of vultures. The reason of this decline was detected after a large gap of time. These vultures were showing signs of renal failure. Later, it was found that the cause of the renal failure was diclofenac (an NSAID), derived from diclofenac treated animal carcasses. These vultures were scavengers of the environment, so their loss posed a massive damage to the ecosystem. Several strategies were devised to decrease the decline of vulture population. These strategies included banning of production and use of diclofenac in veterinary practice, replacement of diclofenac with other NSAIDs like meloxicam which did not pose similar threat to vultures. Captive vulture breeding program was also launched by several countries of South Asian region like India, Nepal and Pakistan to increase the population of vultures which were on the verge of extinction. Such proactive measures were used to counter the deleterious effect of diclofenac on the environment. Pharmacoenvironmentology is new discipline to check the unintended damage to ecosystem, as the environmental threat posed by thousands of drugs is massive.

Keywords: pharmacovigilance, pharmacoenvironmentology, diclofenac, vultures extinction

1. INTRODUCTION

Environmental pharmacology is an emerging specialty of pharmacology. It is defined as the effect of pharmaceuticals and house care products on the environment and ecosystem. It involves the study of gene-environment interaction, drug-environment interaction and toxin-environment interaction, for which specific terminologies have been used very appropriately, i.e., 'Ecogeneology,' 'Ecopharmacology' and 'Ecotoxicology,' respectively (Banjoko 2014).

'Ecopharmacology' (Ecosystem + pharmacology) as a broader term encompasses the entry of both 'pharmaceutics and personal care products (PPCPs)' as well as 'industrial and chemical pollutants (IACPs)' into the environment by any route and at any concentration disturbing the balance of ecology (ecosystem), as a consequence. This impact of PPCPs and

IACPs on environment cannot be a part of Pharmacovigilance activity by virtue of its definition (Rahman et al. 2007).

"Pharmacovigilance is an activity to monitor, detect, assess, understand and prevent any obnoxious adverse drug reactions at therapeutic doses that appear in animal and human beings." The above definition of Pharmacovigilance by WHO is concerned with "therapeutic concentrations." Although, this definition is used in some countries but not in the EU or US where it extends to misuse, abuse, overdose, etc., as well as to the environmental effects (regardless of whether the dose was therapeutic or otherwise). The term 'Pharmacoenvironmentology' deals with the impact of drugs on environment which are given to humans and animals at therapeutic doses.

With the advancement in technology newer and more potent drugs are being manufactured and used on an ever-growing scale in patients for various medical conditions. When a human or animal is given a drug, it may be well or poorly absorbed from the site of administration. Clearly, unabsorbed drug will pass with faeces into the environment. When humans or animals are given drugs they may be metabolized to a greater or lesser extent and thereafter released into the environment as the parent drug or metabolites or a mixture of both. It means that once they are excreted into the environment (direct affection to the environment), they enter food chains and concentrate into larger predators (indirect affection to the human race).

If drugs for human as well as animal use regardless of whether the dose was therapeutic or otherwise enter the environment causing obnoxious reactions subsequent to pharmacotherapy via elimination from living organism, then this concept was defined in a specific domain of Pharmacovigilance or more appropriately a part of Environmental Pharmacovigilance (Rahman 2006). This specific area is now referred as 'PharmacoEnvironmentology' in 2006 (Rahman 2006).

2. DICLOFENAC INDUCED SAGA OF VULTURE EXTINCTION IN SOUTH ASIA

The population of vultures across the Asian subcontinent have shown a rapid decline in the last 15 years and are now on the verge of extinction. Unintentional secondary poisoning of vultures that fed upon carcasses of diclofenac-treated livestock lead to decrease in populations in the Indian subcontinent. The population of vultures in India have declined by 99.9% during last 20 years. Across South Asia tens of millions of vultures have now died. Scientists have warned that three species of Asian vultures could become extinct within 10 years and one, the Oriental white-backed vulture, has lost 99.9 per cent of its population since 1992. According to a study by the Bombay Natural History Society, the oriental white-backed vulture, once thought to be the commonest bird of prey in the world, has lost 99.9% of its population between 1992 and 2007. This makes it the fastest declining wild bird in the history, a demise which is more rapid than that of the 'dodo.' Numbers of long-billed and slender-billed vultures have together fallen by almost 97% in the same period. Populations of the white-rumped vulture, long-billed vulture and slender-billed vultures have declined by more than 90 percent between the years 1992 and 2000. Currently, only 11,000 vultures survive in India. If it continues to decline at this rate, only around 6,000 vultures would be left and finally they may become extinct (Badyal 2008).

Vultures also called "lords of the sky" have a very big role in the Asian eco-system. They dispose off carcasses that would otherwise lead to a significant health risk. Gyps vultures were widely distributed across Asia and Africa.

Gyps indicus found in Indian subcontinent is an Old World vulture in the family Accipitridae, which also includes eagles, kites, buzzards and hawks. It is closely related to the European Griffon Vulture, *G. fulvus*. It breeds on crags or in trees in mountains in Pakistan and India, laying one egg. Birds may form loose colonies. The population is mostly resident. The birds in the eastern part of the range were earlier considered a subspecies.

Now they constitute a separate species, the Slender-billed Vulture Gyps tenuirostris. Previously, both were grouped together as Long-billed Vulture.

The Long-billed Vulture is a typical vulture, with a bald head, very broad wings and short tail feathers. It is smaller and less heavily-built than European Griffon, usually weighing between 5.5 and 6.3 kg (12-13.9 lbs) and measuring 80-100 cm (32-40 in) long and 205-229 cm (81-91 in) across the wings. It is distinguished from that species by its less buff body and wing coverts.

Three vulture species in Asia belonging to the Gyps genus are now critically endangered. These species are the Oriental White-backed Vulture G. bengalensis, Long-billed Vulture G. *indicus* and Slender-billed Vulture G. *tenuirostris*. The loss of these species has lead to massive ecological and social impact in Asia.

The situation on the Indian subcontinent has evolved very rapidly. Concerns for India's vultures were first raised by one of the oldest wildlife conservation organizations of India, Bombay Natural History Society (BNHS) in the late 1990s. Nesting pairs at Keoladeo National Park near Bharatpur, India decreased from 353 in 1987/88 to 20 in 1998-99. No active nests were recorded at the park in either the 1999/2000 or the 2000/01 season. Numbers of Long-billed Vultures also declined from a count of 816 birds in 1985-86 to 25 in 1998-99, with only one bird seen in the 1999-2000 season. Studies reported large numbers of dead adult vultures (73 recorded in 1997/98), suggesting that the decline was related to an increase in mortality rate (Prakash 1999).

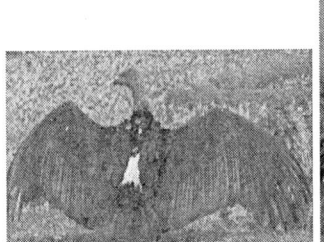 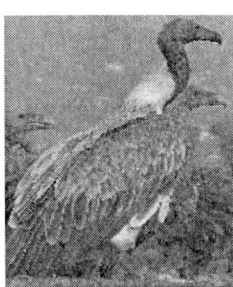 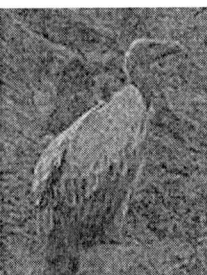

Figure 1. Oriental white-backed Slender-billed Long-billed.

Between 1985-1986 and 1996-1997 the population size of Oriental white-backed vultures declined by an estimated 97% at Keoladeo and in 2003 this colony was extinct. These declines were coupled with high mortality of all age classes. Since the initial surveys, it has been confirmed that these declines have occurred in all regions across India. Some birds appear sick and lethargic for a protracted period before death, often exhibiting a 'neck drooping' posture, characteristic of a vulture that is weak and dehydrated.

In Pakistan, there has been a dramatic decline in the numbers of Oriental white-backed vultures (*Gyps bengalensis*) and in other vulture species. In one area, the decline in the Oriental white-backed vulture has been in the range of 95% since the 1990s (Prakash 1999). There were findings of renal failure and visceral gout in the affected animals. It correlated with findings of high concentrations of the non-steroidal anti-inflammatory drug diclofenac, and the ability of diclofenac to reproduce the effects in the birds. It was hypothesized that the morbidity and mortality in the vultures was due to the animals scavenging on dead livestock which had been treated with diclofenac prior to death. Diclofenac is available as an over the counter veterinary drug in Indian subcontinent and is widely used (Oaks 2004). Attempts to model the toxic effects of diclofenac using domestic poultry have proved unsuccessful (Naidoo 2007). Attempts are now being made to limit the availability of diclofenac (Boston University, School of Public Health, 2002). Drug Controller General of India has notified to ban the use of diclofenac as veterinary medicine in India.

3. Causes of Extinction

After a long interval of time it was possible to find the reason of the disappearanceof the vulture species in India (Hussain 2008). The scientific evidence indicates that diclofenac, a non-steroidal anti-inflammatory drug (NSAIDs) is a major cause of the observed vulture declines (Press Information Bureau, Government of India 2005). After eliminating the classic causes of renal failure, researchers tested the theory that vultures were encountering a toxin while feeding on livestock carcasses (their main food source). Surveys of veterinarians and pharmacists identified diclofenac as a recently introduced and widely used analgesic, known to be toxic to the kidneys of mammals.

In early 2004, The U. S. based Peregrine Fund working in Pakistan found that diclofenac, was responsible for declines in white-rumped vultures in Pakistan. Work by the Bombay Natural History Society, the UK's Royal Society for the Protection of Birds (RSPB), the Zoological Society of London and others extended this work to show diclofenac as the major cause of declines in the vulture declines right across South Asia (Green 2004, 2007).

Diclofenac, is one of the most commonly used painkiller in veterinary practice. It was discovered that the drug's use increased over the same time period as the decline in vultures. It is used to treat lameness and injury - common conditions before a buffalo or cow dies. When these animals die and are eaten by vultures, a single meal will be sufficient to kill the vultures. Experiments show that vultures are highly susceptible to diclofenac and are killed by feeding on the carcass of an animal soon after it has been treated with the normal veterinary dose (Taggart 2006).

Diclofenac causing kidney damage leads to increase in serum uric acid concentrations, visceral gout and death. Acute necrosis of proximal convoluted tubules in these vultures was severe. Glomeruli, DCTs and collecting tubules were comparatively unaffected in the vultures with early lesions. In most vultures, however, lesions were extensive with large urate aggregates obscuring renal architecture. Inflammation was minimal. Excessive uric acid deposition in the organ parenchyma and surface of the organs (visceral gout) was found in vultures with renal failure. Residue testing found diclofenac in all the analysed vultures that had died with visceral gout. Vultures that had died of other causes (including trauma, gunshot and lead poisoning) tested negative for diclofenac residues (Cuthbert 2007).

The vultures that have died in the decline showed kidney damage and uric acid crystals throughout their bodies, but no disease causing microbes or environmental toxins were detected. Vultures that died because of pesticide poisoning or collisions had no uric acid. Analysis of the kidneys from dead vultures with visceral gout has shown diclofenac residues, while no residues were found in other birds. A high proportion of vultures found dead or dying in a much larger area of India and Nepal also have residues of diclofenac and visceral gout, a post-mortem finding such as at Indian Veterinary Research Institute (IVRI), Izzat Nagar (Bareilly, India) that is strongly associated with diclofenac contamination in both species.

Not much is known about the physiological effects of NSAIDs in birds. Diclofenac inhibits prostaglandins (PGs) formation in mammals. The mechanism by which diclofenac induces renal failure in vultures can be through the inhibition of the modulating effect of prostaglandin on angiotensin II-mediated adrenergic stimulation. Renal portal valves open up in response to adrenergic stimulation whisch redirects portal blood to the caudal vena cava and bypasses the kidneys. If diclofenac removes a modulating effect of prostaglandins on the renal portal valves, indiscriminant activation of these valves would redirect the primary nutrient blood supply away from the renal cortex. This would result in ischemic necrosis of the cortical proximal convoluted tubules (Meteyer 2004).

The researchers also gave diclofenac, and meat from animals treated with diclofenac, to non-releasable vultures rescued from nesting colonies. These vultures also died by consuming diclofenac in very small doses, with the same symptoms as the dead, wild vultures. With increase in the dose of the drug, the probability of death increased several folds. Vultures travel large distances to feed on a carcass, so each one gets a small bit of many animals. As few as one in 250 carcasses containing diclofenac at a dose lethal to vultures, would be sufficient to cause the observed decline in vulture numbers (30% per year). So even small-scale use of the drug can have catastrophic consequences.

Diclofenac was found to be lethal to vultures at 10 percent of the therapeutic mammalian dose. Tissue residues in livestock treated at the labeled dose rate were sufficient to cause gout and death in vultures. These findings, coupled with the high incidence of visceral gout in wild vultures found dead in Pakistan, India and Nepal confirm that diclofenac is the primary cause of the Asian vulture decline. Analyses indicate that the level of diclofenac contamination found in carcasses of domesticated ungulates in 2004-2005 was sufficient to account for the observed rapid decline of the oriental white-backed vulture in India.

Diclofenac is an anti-inflammatory and analgesic. The name is derived from its chemical name: 2-(2, 6-dichloranilino) phenylacetic acid. In the United Kingdom, India, and the United States, it is supplied as either the sodium or potassium salt, in China most often as the sodium salt, while in some other countries only as the potassium salt. Diclofenac is available as a generic drug in various formulations. Over the counter (OTC) use is approved in some countries for minor problems.

Mortality in vultures was also found following treatment with ibuprofen and phenylbutazone. NSAID toxicity was reported for raptors, storks, cranes and owls, suggesting that the potential conservation impact of NSAIDs may extend beyond Gyps vultures and could be significant for New World vultures. Diclofenac is widely used globally and could present a risk to Gyps species from other regions too.

4. ADVERSE CONSEQUENCES

While the extinction of vultures may not strike the same cord as other cuter creatures, they play a vital role in the Asian eco-system. Vultures are keystone species and their declines are having adverse effects upon other wildlife, domestic animals and humans. This imposes a heightened risk of diseases that threaten human life and welfare.

In India, vultures have traditionally disposed of carcasses in cities, villages and the countryside, reducing the risk of disease and helping with sanitation. With the vultures gone, carcasses are likely to take much longer to be stripped, increasing the risk to health. The massive vulture disappearances had terrible consequences throughout India (Taggart 2007). With no vultures to eat cattle carcasses (which are just dumped when the cows die), other predators have filled the gap. Feral dogs are filling the scavenging void, and their growing numbers also increase risks to human health and safety. Since they are carriers of rabies.

Populations of feral dogs have increased massively in recent past with an increase of 5.5 million more dogs to the streets. As per a report published in the journal Ecological Economics suggests this massive increase in feral dogs has led to dramatic increase in attacks on humans numbering in millions and caused atleast 47,300 human deaths from rabies. Indian experts have recorded a sharp rise in the number of feral dogs as they fill the gap in the food chain, and with that an increase in the number of cases of rabies and other diseases. The population of rats have also increased, and that's always a harbinger of diseases to come (Badyal 2008).

5. Strategies to Check Extinction

Halting and reversing the decline in vulture population is one of the most urgent conservation priorities. The solution to this problem requires commitment by governments and pharmaceutical industry. As per conservationists, the birds can only be saved by banning the use of diclofenac and setting up a network of captive breeding centres (Swan 2005).

Although, manufacture of the drug has been outlawed in India since 2006 however it remains easily available. Farmers and vets simply switched to the human form of diclofenac despite an effective and safer alternative drug being available. Measures that make veterinary and human diclofenac less easy to use are crucial if we are to save these birds. Steps to make meloxicam, which is as effective to make it more widely available are just as important.

Vulture populations are already at critically low levels. On the 11th of May 2006, the Drug Controller General (India) ordered the withdrawal of all licenses granted for the manufacture of diclofenac for veterinary use within India. Although the Indian Government banned the veterinary use of diclofenac, this obviously needs to be implemented and properly enforced before vulture numbers can even start to recover. Diclofenac was also banned in Pakistan and Nepal in 2006, after Indian Government's initiative.

5.1. Meloxicam - The Diclofenac Replacement

The drug meloxicam is safer for the vultures at the likely range of levels they would be exposed to in the wild. The Drug Controller General of India had issued a directive to phase out veterinary Diclofenac and replace it with Meloxicam. Meloxicam, which is similar to diclofenac in its effectiveness for treating livestock, has recently become available for veterinary use in India and could easily be used in place of diclofenac. This recommendation was based on extensive acute safety studies in the African White-backed vulture (*Gyps africanus*), which evaluated worst case scenarios of maximum intake based on a once in three day feeding pattern. There were no reported mortalities for the NSAID meloxicam, which was administered to over 700 birds from 60 species. The relative safety of meloxicam supported by a number of studies indicates the suitability of this NSAID to replace diclofenac in Asia. Aceclofenac in caltle is metabolized into diclofenac, which will again harm the vultures (Galligan 2016).

5.2. Environmental Risk Assessment for Diclofenac

Many models were proposed to screen the effect of PPCPs in Aquatic and Terrestrial Environment (Rahman 2018, Naidoo 2007). Uptake and Biological Effects of Environmentally Relevant Concentrations of the Nonsteroidal Anti-inflammatory Pharmaceutical Diclofenac in Rainbow Trout (*Oncorhynchus mykiss*) is thoroughly studied by Mehinto (Mehinto 2010).

Preclinical safety testing has not been well established for avian species unlike for mammalian and environmental toxicity, Hasan IZ et al.

(Hasan 2018) put forward a question if there was a preclinical model that could have predicted the toxic effect of the drug. To test the acute toxic potential of pesticides in birds under Organisation for Economic Co-operation and Development (OECD) guidelines (guideline 223), three avian species were exposed to the drug. Exposed Japanese quails (Coturnix japonica) and Muscovy ducks (Cairina moschata) had shown similar clinical signs and pathology to those previously reported in vultures, i.e., hyperuricemia, depression, death, visceral gout and nephrosis. However, exposed domestic pigeons (Columba livia domestica) were insensitive. Following a pharmacokinetic analysis, the drug was well absorbed and distributed in the pigeons with a half-life below 6 h. A toxicokinetic evaluation in quails showed poisoning was due to metabolic constraint, with a half-life and mean residence time above 6 h and 8 h respectively resulting in death. Toxicity seen in the ducks was however not related to metabolic constraint but hyperuricemia as metabolism was rapid [half-life (1-2 h) and mean residence time (2-3 h)] irrespective of survival or death. Despite succumbing to diclofenac, the established oral median lethal dose (LD_{50}) of 405.42 mg/kg and 189.92 mg/kg in Japanese quails and Muscovy ducks respectively from this study were substantially higher than those reported for Gyps vultures (0.098 mg/kg) which is as a result of the rapid elimination of the drug from the body in the former species. More importantly, it suggests that these species are not suitable as surrogates for non-steroidal anti-inflammatory drug toxicity testing and that the toxicity of diclofenac in vultures is idiosyncratic most likely as a result of species specific metabolism (Hassan 2018).

5.3. Captive Vulture Breeding Program

Captive breeding program is the most important tool in the fight against the extinction of vultures. Three captive breeding centres housing the three species under impending extinction have been built across India. One is in Harayana housing 120 vultures, the second in West Bengal holds 52 vultures and the third in Assam holds 10 vultures. Few other centres have been built in south Asian countries like Nepal and Pakistan. These centres aim to hold viable populations of all three species. The Vulture Care Centre at Pinjore, Haryana, operated by the Bombay Natural History Society now holds good numbers of Indian and White-rumped Vultures, and received its first Slender-billed Vultures in early 2006. A further centre to house Slender-billed Vultures at Rajabhatkhawa, outside the Buxa Tiger Reserve in West Bengal, has also now been completed, receiving its first occupants in early 2006. Other centres, in association with Zoological Society of London (ZSL) and WWF-Pakistan are planned in Nepal and Pakistan, respectively.

Conservationists want to bring vultures into captivity as rapidly as possible to establish conservation breeding populations. Birds should then be released back into the wildlife when vulture populations are breeding and the environment is effectively free from diclofenac.

A study of 11 of Nepal's 75 administrative districts by Bird Conservation Nepal (BCN, BirdLife in Nepal) finds that the use of diclofenac has dropped by 90 per cent since 2006. The work by BCN and its partners, notably the Nepalese government (Department of Drug Administrative and Department of National Parks and Wildlife Conservation) is worth to be appreciable in this direction. BCN is working collaboratively for a complete phasing out of diclofenac and other harmful NSAID drugs from the market. Support has come not only from conservation organisations such as the Royal Society for the Protection of Birds (RSPB) (Birdlife in the UK), ZSL and WWF, but also from local veterinary and para-veterinary practitioners, local pharmacists, pharmaceuticals distributors associations and local communities. In ten districts of western Nepal including Chitwan, BCN has replaced half a million rupees ($8,000) worth of diclofenac with the safe and equally effective alternative drug, meloxicam. Conservationists in Nepal have opened an eatery for the unlovely scavengers. It is in the Nawalparasi district in southwest Nepal. The niche 'restaurant' has been operating for a little over a year. Since then, the population of the vultures has almost doubled in the region. What is special about the restaurant is that it ensures the birds get food that is free of Diclofenac. A number of volunteers and two full-time employees working for the eatery collect sick cows and care for them till they die. Then they physically cart them to the open field that serves as the restaurant for these birds. In collaboration with a number of government and non-governmental agencies, over the last five years BCN has also conducted a massive conservation-awareness program throughout Nepal, highlighting the importance of vultures in maintaining balanced ecosystems.

There are early indications that the mortality of the vulture population has been reduced but not stopped. Chris Bowden, the RSPB's vulture-program manager, said, "The Indian government is to be congratulated on taking this huge step that we have working towards ever since the discovery that diclofenac was such an acute problem."

All said and done, and despite the introduction of the safe drug Meloxicam, Diclofenac is still being used in India and Nepal (Cuthbert 2016). At the Rani Vulture breeding and conservation site in Guwahati (India), for instance, the population of Gyp vultures is fast disappearing. Field workers and researchers on the ground attribute it to the use of Diclofenac. Wildlife enthusiasts are launching aggressive campaigns to enforce the ban on the use of Diclofenac still widely available in India. Other groups are focusing on providing safe food for vultures. They do look ugly, but they are certainly essential for the hygiene of our community.

Acknowledgments

We thank the Centre for Safety and Rational Use of Indian Systems of Medicine (CSRUISM), Ibn Sīnā Academy of Medieval Medicine and Sciences (IAMMS), Aligarh, India, for providing resource materials in writing the above paper.

REFERENCES

Anonymous 2002, 'Pharmaceuticals in environment,' *Health Effects Review*, An official journal of Department of Environmental Health, Boston University School of Public Health, 1-3.

Badyal D 2008, 'Drug Induced Saga of Vulture Extinction in India,' In: Rahman SZ, Shahid M & Gupta V Eds. *An Introduction to Environmental Pharmacology*. Ibn Sina Academy, Aligarh, India, 177-186.

Bosun Banjoko 2014 'Environmental Pharmacology - An Overview,' *Pharmacology and Therapeutics*, InTech.

Cuthbert, R., Parry-Jones, J., Green, R. E., Pain, D. J. 2007, 'NSAIDs and scavenging birds: potential impacts beyond Asia's critically endangered vultures,' *Environ. Int.*, 33: 759-65.

Galligan, T. H., Taggart, M. A., Cuthbert, R. J., Svobodova, D., Chipangura, J., Alderson, D., Prakash, V. M., and Naidoo 2016, V Metabolism of aceclofenac in cattle to vulture-killing diclofenac. *Conservation Biology*, 30: 1122-1127.

Green, R. E., Newton, I., Shultz, S., Andrew, A., Cunningham, Gilbert M., Deborah J., Pain & Prakash V., 2004, 'Diclofenac poisoning as a cause of vulture population declines across the Indian subcontinent,' *Journal of Applied Ecology* 41, 793-800.

Green R. E., Taggart M. A., Senacha K. R., Raghavan B., Pain D. J., Jhala Y., Cuthbert R. 2007, 'Rate of decline of the oriental white-backed vulture population in India estimated from a survey of diclofenac residues in carcasses of ungulates,' *Biol. Lett.* 3: 90-3.

Hassan, I. Z., Duncan, N., Adawaren, E. O., Naidoo, V. 2018, 'Could the environmental toxicity of diclofenac in vultures been predictable if preclinical testing methodology were applied?' *Environ. Toxicol. Pharmacol.* 64:181-186.

Irtaza, Hussain, M. Zargham, Khan, Ahrar, Khan, Ijaz, Javed & M. Kashif Saleemi 2008 'Toxicological effects of diclofenac in four avian species,' *Avian Pathology* 37 (3): 315-321.

Mehinto, Alvine C., Hill, Elizabeth M., and Tyler Charles R., 2010, Uptake and Biological Effects of Environmentally Relevant Concentrations of the Nonsteroidal Anti-inflammatory Pharmaceutical Diclofenac in Rainbow Trout (Oncorhynchus mykiss). *Environmental Science & Technology* 44 (6), 2176-2182.

Meteyer CU, Rideout BA, Gilbert M, Shivaprasad HL, Oaks JL 2004 'Pathology and proposed pathophysiology of diclofenac poisoning in free-living and experimentally exposed oriental white-backed vultures (Gyps bengalensis),' *Proc. Biol. Sci.* 271 Suppl. 6:S458-60.

Naidoo V, Wolter K, Cromarty AD, Bartels P, Bekker L, McGaw L 2007, 'The pharmacokinetics of meloxicam in vultures,' *PLoS ONE* 2:e686.

Oaks JL, Gilbert M, Virani MZ, Watson RT, Meteyer CU, Rideout BA 2004, 'Diclofenac residues as the cause of vulture population decline in Pakistan,' *Nature* 427: 630-3.

Press Information Bureau, Government of India (2005-05-16). Saving vultures from extinction, press release (http://pib.nic.in/release/release.asp?relid=9303. Retrieved on 2006-05-12).

Rahman SZ, Khan RA, Kumar V, Misbahuddin M 2007 'Pharmaco-environmentology - A Component of Pharmacovigilance,' *BMC Environmental Health* 6:20.

Rahman SZ 2018, 'Need of Designing Model for Screening of PPCPs (Ecopharmacology) and Therapeutic Drugs (Pharmacoenvironmentology) in Aquatic and Terrestrial Environment,' *IABCR* 4(3):100-5.

Rahman SZ 2006, 'Impact of Human Medicines on Environment - A New Emerging Problem,' *Population Envis.* 3(2):3-4.

Richard J Cuthbert, Mark A Taggart, Mohini Saini, Anil Sharma, Asit Das, Mandar D Kulkarni, Parag Deori, Sachin Ranade, Rohan N Shringarpure, Toby H Galligan and Rhys E Green 2016, 'Continuing mortality of vultures in India associated with illegal veterinary use of diclofenac and a potential threat from nimesulide,' *Oryx* 50 (1): 104-112.

Swan G, Naidoo V, Cuthbert R, Green RE, Pain DJ, Swarup D 2005, 'Removing the threat of diclofenac to critically endangered Asian vultures,' *J. Wildl. Dis.* 41: 707-16.

Taggart M. A., Senacha K. R., Green R. E., Jhala Y. V., Raghavan B, Rahmani AR 2006, 'Diclofenac residues in carcasses of domestic ungulates available to vultures in India,' *PLoS Biol.* 4:e66.

Taggart, M. A., Cuthbert, R., Das, D., Sashikumar, C., Pain, D. J., Green R. E., Feltrer, Y., Shultz, S., Cunningham, A. A., Meharg, A. A. 2007, 'Diclofenac disposition in Indian cow and goat with reference to *Gyps* vulture population declines,' *Environmental Pollution* 147 (1): 60-65.

V Prakash 1999, 'Status of vultures in Keoladeo National Park, Bharatpur, Rajasthan with special reference to population crash in *Gyps* species,' *J. Bombay Natural History Society*, 96: 365-378.

V Naidoo, N Duncan, L Bekker, G Swan 2007, 'Validating the domestic fowl as a model to investigate the pathophysiology of diclofenac in Gyps vultures,' *Environmental Toxicology and Pharmacology* 24 (3): 260-266.

In: Environmental Pharmacology of Diclofenac ISBN: 978-1-53617-466-3
Editor: Eugenia Yiannakopoulou © 2020 Nova Science Publishers, Inc.

Chapter 3

ENVIRONMENTAL TOXICITY OF DICLOFENAC

Francis Orata[*], *PhD*

Department of Pure and Applied Chemistry,
Masinde Muliro University of Science and Technology,
Kakamega, Kenya

ABSTRACT

Diclofenac is a widely used medicine with a potent analgesic, anti-inflammatory, and antipyretic actions. As a result, it is approved for treatment of rheumatoid arthritis, osteoarthritis, ankylosing spondylitis, dysmenorrhea, ocular inflammation and actinic keratosis among other health conditions. However, diclofenac is banned for veterinary use in many countries due to its discovered toxicity to animals. Studies have demonstrated that diclofenac can elicit responses in aquatic organisms at relatively low concentrations. Diclofenac presence has been detected and quantified throughout the various environmental matrices. Among the matrices where quantifiable levels of diclofenac have been obtained are

---

[*] Corresponding Author's Email: fraora@yahoo.com.

drinking water, groundwater, sediment and wastewater which is from wastewater treatment plants. Theses contaminants presence in environmental matrices acts as a source or discharge point of diclofenac pollution to non-target organisms. As a consequence, unmetabolized form of diclofenac may enter the food chain and thus increase the potential to course adverse health effects posed to human and other organisms. In Human, diclofenac consumption has been associated with side effects on the cardiovascular, gastrointestinal, hepatic and renal systems among others. To date, most control policy and measures on diclofenac are informed by its acute toxicity. However, chronic toxicity, synergistic or antagonistic effects of diclofenac molecule but its metabolites and products of their reaction with other environmental molecules present, should inform the future policy and directives. The aim of this chapter is to discuss the environmental toxicity of diclofenac. The chapter will also report the on the occurrence of diclofenac in various environmental matrices and evaluate the risk they pose to non-target organisms.

Keywords: diclofenac, environmental toxicity, environmental levels, fate, risks

1. INTRODUCTION

Diclofenac is an anti-inflammatory drug (NSAID) and an antiphlogistic active pharmaceutical ingredient that is administered via oral ingestion or by dermal absorption. It is categorized as an extended-release tablet. Structurally, diclofenac sodium is a benzeneacetic acid derivative with a chemical name is 2- ((2, 6-dichlorophenyl) amino) benzeneacetic acid, monosodium salt. The molecular weight is 318.13 and molecular formula is $C_{14}H_{10}C_{12}NNaO_2$. The structural formula is shown in Figure 1 as either a K^+ or Na^+ salt. The main difference between the two is that diclofenac potassium is absorbed into the body more quickly than diclofenac sodium.

The chemical CAS number is 15307-86-5 15307-79-6 and has an EU number, 239-348-5 239-346-4 (for diclofenac sodium salt). Commercially, proprietary names of pharmaceuticals containing diclofenac or diclofenac sodium salt are: Acoflam; Arthrotec; Cataflam; Dicloflex; Diclomax; Diclotard; Diclovol; Diclozip; Econac; Flamatak; Flamrase; Flexotard;

Isclofen; Lofensaid; Motifene; Pennsaid; Rheumatac; Rhumalgan; Slofenac; Solaraze; Volraman; Volsaid; Voltaren(e); Voltarol among others not mentioned in this chapter. A quick action is useful where immediate pain relief is required, and a prolonged action is more useful in reducing inflammation. Some brands of diclofenac also contain a medicine called misoprostol. The brands proprietary names Arthrotec and Misofen are prescribed for arthritis. Misoprostol helps to protect the stomach against irritation which can be caused by taking diclofenac over a period of time.

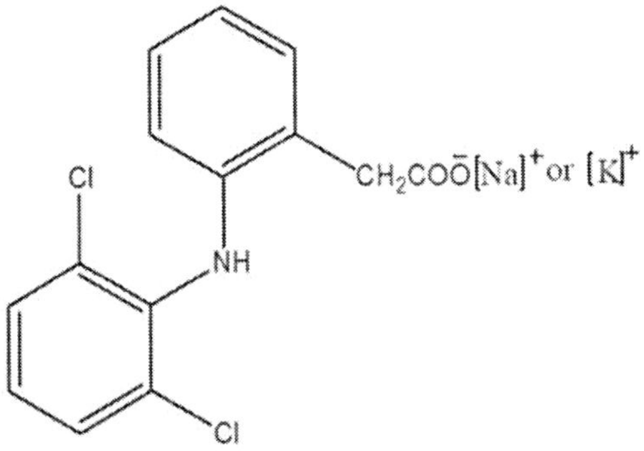

Figure 1. Structure of diclofenac, as a sodium or potassium salt.

1.1. Physical and Chemical Characteristics

There are varying physical chemical characteristics that influence pharmacokinetics, diclofenac distribution and fate in environment matrices, such as water solubility, vapour pressure, partition coefficients especially for water (Kow) and organic carbon (Koc). Organic carbon – water partition coefficient (K_{OC}) at various pHs which greatly influences adsorption 1450 mLg^{-1}, 874 mLg^{-1}, 2.30 mLg^{-1}, 1 mLg^{-1} at pH = 1, pH = 4, pH = 7, pH = 8 - 10, calculated, respectively (ACS Daten Bank, 2004). Various studies reported the following Koc values for diclofenac; 47 - 1310 LKg^{-1} for sludge (Ternes, 2004), 61.7 – 83.2 cm^{3}g^{-1} for soil (Chefetz, 2008) and log Koc 2.45 - 3.74 for sediments (Scheytt, 2005). Diclofenac molecule is a lipophilic and has a carboxylic group, which has the weakly acidic characteristic and with a seemingly high octanol - water partition (Avdeef et al., 1998). The Octanol-water partition coefficient (Log Kow) for diclofenac was reported to as 4.02, with the lipophilicity measurement (Log P) calculated as 3.28 ± 0.36 (Syracuse Science Center, 2002). Bioconcentration factors (BCFs) are used to relate pollutant residues in aquatic organisms to the pollutant concentration in ambient waters. Studies have examined the bioaccumulation of pharmaceuticals and their fate in the water and aquatic organisms. For example, the bioaccumulation factor (BCF) for diclofenac measured in fish were reported over a 12 days period in plasma was found to be 2.5 - 29 (Fick, 2010). BCF measured in Mussel, (*Mytilus edulis trossulus*), of 1 μgl^{-1} exposure for whole body was 180 (Ericson et al., 2010).

Since 1990 and following the incidences that resulted to the catastrophic declines of >95% vultures (*Gyps indicus* and *Gyps tenuirostris*,) that is associated with diclofenac toxicity to non-target organisms (Oaks et al., 2004; Oaks and Watson 2011), and the subsequent listing of these vultures as endangered, there has been a raising international concern on diclofenac adverse effects that can result from its continual use and detection as a pollutant in the environment (Prakash et al., 2003). Diclofenac was proposed to be added to the priority list, but members of European Parliament rejected the purpose of establish an EQS for pharmaceuticals. The Commission also proposed a watch-list mechanism for gathering monitoring data to support future reviews of the list (BIO Intelligence Service, 2013). There is need for more research and discussion on the use and the adverse effects of diclofenac on human and non-target organisms that is based on the occurrence and levels of diclofenac in various environmental matrices.

2. Environmental Levels and Fate

All over the world, several studies have revealed that drugs are emerging environmental contaminants that are widely spread in effluents of wastewater treatment plants, in freshwater and marine surface waters, and in ground and drinking water (Fent et al., 2006; Kimosop et al., 2016; Benotti et al., 2009; Weber et al., 2014). Pharmaceutical active compounds are found in the environment in the ngL^{-1} to $\mu g\ L^{-1}$ levels (Zhang et al., 2013). These low concentrations have made pharmaceutical compounds undetectable in various environmental matrices, until recently when more advancement in modern analytical techniques detection limits have been improved (Santos et al., 2010). The presence of diclofenac in water can be explained in terms of both their excretion through urine and faeces in unmetabolized forms and their inefficient removal from water treatment systems. German Advisory Council on the Environment (GACE) reported diclofenac levels exceeding 50 tonnes/year annual consumption levels, together with other analgesic drugs like paracetamol and the antibiotic sulphamethoxazole or amoxicillin (GACE, 2007). A report in 2008 estimated the overall yearly worldwide consumption of diclofenac as a human and veterinary pharmaceutical drug to be >1000 tons/year (Zhang et al., 2008). These quantities have a potential or contaminating the environment is proper disposal of diclofenac and other pharmaceutical substances are not followed. Diclofenac has been detected in wastewater treatment plants in a number of countries. The poor adsorption of diclofenac to activated sludge and resistance to biodegradation means its removal rate from wastewater is generally low (measured at between 21 and 40%) (Zhang et al., 2013; Kimura et al., 2007; Johnson et al., 2013; Gardner et al., 2013). Because most wastewater treatment plants are unable to remove diclofenac, it has been detected in groundwater, surface water, and wastewater effluents, as well as in drinking water at concentrations ranging between ngL^{-1} and μgL^{-1} (Chen et al., 2014; Memmert et al., 2013; Langenhoff et al., 2013). Figure 2 show the discharge points and sources of diclofenac introduction and distribution into the aquatic environment. Diclofenac was detected in almost all surveys of surface waters with concentration levels in the ngL^{-1} range (Fent at al., 2006). Results from the analyses of waste water treatment plants (LUBW, 2014) show that diclofenac detection in the influent and effluent exceeded the proposed Environmental Quality Standards (EQSs), of $4 \times 10^{-4}\ \mu g\ L^{-1}$. Johnson et al.

(2014) used a geographic based water model to predict the environmental concentrations of the three watch list pharmaceuticals, 17α-ethinylestradiol (EE2), 17β-estradiol (E2), and diclofenac throughout European rivers. The study predicted an increase in of these pharmaceutical compounds in the environment. Studies have shown that diclofenac residue in environmental matrices such as sediment can be ingested by microorganisms and thus giving an insight on the fate of diclofenac in the environment. Karlsson et al., (2016) reported the ingestion of diclofenac in sediment-dwelling worm *Lumbriculus variegatus*. In the study, the biota sediment accumulation factors (BSAF), based on uptake of labeled carbon ^{14}C, for feeding worms was 0.5.

Calculations of predicted environmental concentrations (PNEC) are made according European Chemical Bureau, Institute for Health and Consumer Protection, (2008) using the following equation;

$$PNEC = \frac{X}{Risk\ asssessment\ factor},$$

where X is LC_{50}, EC_{50}, IC_{50} or NOEC

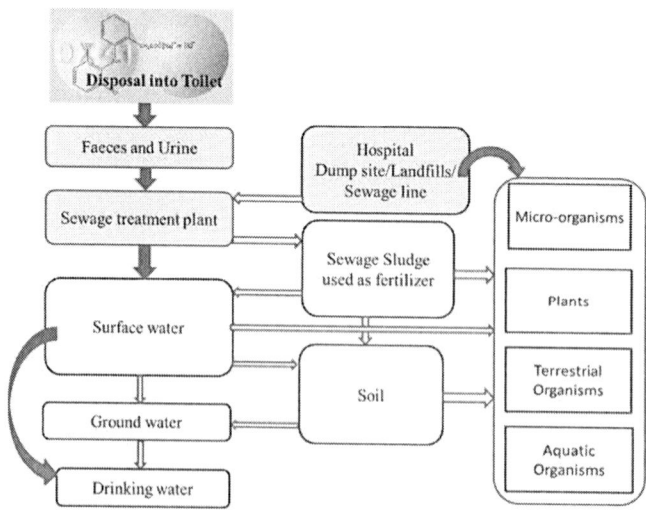

Figure 2. Sources and the cycle of diclofenac in abiotic and biotic facilities and general environment.

Table 1. Enviromental Concentrations of Diclofenac and Calculated Predicted No-Effect Concentration (PNEC) in various environmental matrices

Compartment	Location and setting	Measured environmental concentration	Reference
Freshwater	Germany, Maximum of the average by station (n=72), year 2008	0.71 µgL^{-1}	Umweltbundesamt, 2010
	Germany, Maximum of analyses, year 2008	1.7 µgL^{-1}	Umweltbundesamt, 2010
	Maximum environmental concentration	1200 µgL^{-1}	KNAPPE, 2008
Marine waters	Estuary of the river Elbe, (coastal and/or transitional)	6.2 µgL^{-1}	Weigel 2002
	UK estuaries	Max. 195 µgL^{-1} and median of < 8 µgL^{-1}	Thomas 2004
	Canada Atlantic coast, receiving untreated sewage	Max. 6 µgL^{-1}; median: 3 ng.l	Comeau 2008
Wastewater	6 in WWTP influent, Germany	Bdl – 6.9 µgL^{-1} Mean 1.8	LUBW, 2014
	6 in WWTP effluent, Germany	0.065 – 2.8 µgL^{-1} Mean 1.0	LUBW, 2014
	Germany, WWTP effluent	4.7 µgL^{-1}	Heberer 2002
		0.25 – 5.45 µgL^{-1}	Andreozzi 2003
	Germany, WWTP effluent	2.1 µgL^{-1}	Ternes, 2001
	Germany, WWTP effluent	1.59 µgL^{-1}	Stan and Heberer, 1997
	Germany, WWTP effluent	1.03 µgL^{-1}	Heberer et al., 2002
	Germany, WWTP effluent	1.2 µgL^{-1}	Ternes, 2001
	France	0.29 µgL^{-1}	Ferrari et al 2004
	France	0.41 µgL^{-1}	Ferrari et al 2004
Sediment	max in Germany	400 ng L^{-1}	Ferreira da Silva, 2011
	(Greifensee lake, Switzerland)	nd	Buser, 1998
	Valencian Community, Spain	nd	Vazquez-Roig, 2010
Biota	Fish Plasma Model: In plasma of rainbow trout exposed to sewage effluents	12 ng/ml at one site, below limit of detection (< 3 ng/ml) at two other sites.	Brown 2007
Calculated Predicted No-Effect Concentration (PNEC)	France and Germany Blue-green alga PNEC$_{acute}$	10 000 ng L^{-1}	Roche, 2012
		14.5 mg L^{-1}	Ferrari et al., 2004
		20 mg L^{-1}	Ferrari et al., 2005
	France and Germany Crustacean PNEC$_{chronic}$	6 000 ng L^{-1}	Kümmerer, 2008
		100 ng L^{-1}	Bergmann, 2011
Surface water	German rivers	200 – 500 ngL^{-1}	Mompelat, 2009 Ter Laak, 2010) GACE, 2007
	Hérault watershed, France	2 ng L^{-1}	Mompelat, 2009
	French rivers	2 ng L^{-1}	Vulliet, 2011
Groundwater	German groundwater	60 – 400 ng L^{-1}	GACE, 2007
	French groundwater	400 ng L^{-1}	KNAPPE, 2008

PNEC$_{acute}$ = predicted no-effected concentration derived from acute tests (excluding bacteria); PNEC$_{chronic}$ = predicted no-effect concentration derived from chronic tests (excluding bacteria); KNAPPE = Knowledge and Need Assessment on Pharmaceutical Products in Environmental Waters.

The calculation of PNEC requires integrating the information on predicted amounts of pollutant used and specific removal rates in a wastewater treatment plants or surface waters. The results are then analyzed on the value of PEC on standard value of concentrations of above 10 ngL^{-1}. Some calculated PNEC values from previous studies are shown in Table 1.

The European Commission sub-group on review of the priority substances list (2011) reported that an indicative quality standard of 0.007 µgL^{-1} was calculated for diclofenac, with an accumulation factor of 1000 and an extrapolated whole body bioconcentration factor (BCF) of 147 for fish.

The quality standards of the freshwater ecosystem is considered to be critical for the derivation of an environmental quality standard (EQS), in view of the uncertainty regarding the calculation from the biota EQS of the corresponding water EQS. EQS for diclofenac in freshwater and saltwater are 0.1 µgL^{-1} and 0.01 µgL^{-1} respectively. The EQS for pelagic communities in freshwater and saltwater is 0.1µgL^{-1} and 0.01 µgL^{-1} respectively, and for predators (secondary poisoning) is 1 µgkg$^{-1}_{\text{biota ww}}$ and 0.007 µgL^{-1} for fresh and marine water predators.

2.1. Diclofenac Degradation

Generally, diclofenac is poorly biodegradable which often translates into low elimination rates from the environment and also during biological wastewater treatment. Although diclofenac was observed to be only partially biodegraded in all enrichment cultures (Sari et al., 2014), enhanced elimination can be achieved by bioaugmentation. Microbial communities that are able to degrade diclofenac, were studied by Bessa et al., (2017) where Strain *Brevibacterium sp.* was found to be able to biodegrade 35% of 10 mgL^{-1} of diclofenac as a sole carbon source (More information is needed to gain more information about the deconjugation processes and biotic and abiotic transformation and the nature of transformation products (Vieno, and Sillanpää, 2014). Gröning et al., (2007) obtained a Half-life time (DT$_{50}$) of 5.5 - 18.6 days depletion from a fixed-bed column bioreactor filled with sediment under aerobic conditions thus showing a significant biodegradation. In the study, *p*-benzoquinone imine of 5-hydroxydiclofenac was obtained as a major metabolite.

Results for photolysis showed that rapid degradation of diclofenac to a level <1% of the initial concentration after 4 days exposure to sunlight (DT$_{50}$ < 4days) (Buser, 1998), DT$_{50}$ = 2.4 days (in salt and organic-free water, 50° N in winter) (Andreozzi, 2003) and DT50 = 39 min (in natural water and Milli-Q water, 45° N in summer) (Packer, 2003). Indirect photolysis occurs in the presence of strong oxidant species, such as hydroxyl radicals and singlet oxygen. Hydroxyl radical-mediated photolysis of diclofenac was reported by Andreozzi et al., (2003) and Packer et al., (2003). Few studies have shown an increase in toxicity of the photoproducts of anti-inflammatory drugs (Isidori et al. 2006). Advanced oxidation processes by means of combining different highly oxidizing agents, such as H_2O_2/ozone or UV/ozone, can provide the best removal rate for diclofenac (99.9%) (Jjemba, 2008). Other studies have been done on electro-oxidation of pharmaceutical active ingredients. For example, Sifuna et al., (2016) did comparative studies in electrochemical degradation of diclofenac in water by using various electrodes and phosphate and sulfate supporting electrolytes. In the study, the cyclic voltammetric studies show that diclofenac and sulfamethoxazole are electrochemically active PhACs as demonstrated by the increase in the oxidation peaks of the PhACs with increasing concentration. The results showed that Na_2SO_4 was 15 - 30% more efficient in the electrochemical degradation of both diclofenac and sulfamethoxazole on Platinum and Carbon electrodes than potassium phosphate buffer. The rate of mineralization of the diclofenac at Platinum anode was found to be better than on the carbon anode. The kinetics study shows that the degradation diclofenac follows the second order reaction with correlation coefficient above 0.9. The second-order degradation kinetics indicated that the rate-determining step in the degradation could be a chemical process, thus suggesting the active involvement of electrolyte radical species in the degradation of diclofenac and sulfamethoxazole. The major products expected from electro-oxidation process are simple molecules which are often in gaseous state (Sifuna et al., 2016). In a similar study by Zhaoqi et al., (2017) on electrochemical degradation of diclofenac for pharmaceutical wastewater treatment, it was observed that the electrochemical degradation of diclofenac was achieved employing BDD and Ta/PbO anodes. Specifically, the oxidation of diclofenac was promoted by hydroxyl radicals generated via the oxidation of water on the surface of BDD and Ta/PbO. The degradation efficiency of diclofenac on the Ta/PbO anode increased with an increasing current density and temperature (Zhaoqi et al., 2017). Perez-Estrada et al., (2005) studied the photo-fenton degradation of diclofenac by advanced oxidation processes (AOPs). Results obtained show rapid and complete oxidation of diclofenac after 60 min and total mineralization (disappearance of dissolved organic carbon, DOC) after 100 min of exposure to sunlight.

3. ADVERSE ECOLOGICAL EFFECTS AND TOXICITY

Adverse environmental effects have been observed in other organisms, which are mainly within the aquatic ecology. Cuklev et al., (2011), investigated global hepatic gene expression together with bioconcentration in blood plasma and liver of rainbow trout (*Oncorhynchus mykiss*) exposed to waterborne diclofenac, in order to relate internal exposure to a pharmacological interaction. The study reported that at the highest exposure concentration (81.5 µgL^{-1}), the fish plasma concentration reached approximately 88% of the human therapeutic levels (C_{max}) after two weeks, and found extensive effects on hepatic gene expression at this concentration, with some genes found to be regulated down to the lowest exposure concentration tested (1.6 µg L^{-1}), corresponding to a plasma concentration approximately 1.5% of the human C_{max}. After chronic exposure, several authors observed histopathological effects in trout species at relatively low concentrations around 1.0 to 5.0 mg/L (Mehinto et al., 2010) as opposed to acute exposure (Lee et al., 2011). Praskova et al., (2014) investigate effects of subchronic exposure to sublethal levels of diclofenac on growth, oxidative stress, and histopathological changes in in Zebrafish (*Danio rerio*) and observed a significant decrease in the fish growth caused by diclofenac concentrations of 30 and 60 mg L^{-1}. These findings induced a public concern regarding a risk of diclofenac to fish populations. A study by Memmert et al., (2013), on chronic toxicity and bioconcentration in fish, obtained a bioconcentration factor (BCF) in rainbow trout below 10, demonstrating no relevant bioconcentration of diclofenac in fish. In the study (Memmert et al., 2013), the authors considered consider the moderately reduced growth of zebrafish that was observed due to exposure to concentrations of up to 320 µg/L not to be a repeatable and treatment-related effect of diclofenac. Thus, diclofenac was considered to have no adverse effect on both fish species up to 320 µg/L.

A significant bioconcentration of diclofenac was measured in some fish organs (Schwaiger et al., 2004). These findings of chronic toxicity and bioconcentration in fish are currently the main basis for many stakeholders to conclude that even the low concentrations of diclofenac measured in surface waters present a high risk to the environment. Guiloski et al. (2015) evaluated the effects of diclofenac and dexamethasone in male fish *Hoplias malabaricus* after trophic exposure. The results obtained indicated that diclofenac and dexamethasone reduced the levels of testosterone in male fish of *Hoplias malabaricus* and caused liver oxidative stress to *Hoplias malabaricus*. The study also reported that Anti-inflammatories diclofenac and dexamethasone may have negative impacts in aquatic organisms (Guiloski et al., 2015). Schmitt-Jansen et al., (2007) reported several photo-transformation products that resulted from diclofenac exposure to natural sunlight, in laboratory assays as well as in natural water systems. Toxicological experiments were done by the exposed to natural sunlight to synchronized cultures of the unicellular chlorophyte (*Scenedesmus vacuolatus*). The results showed inhibition of the algal reproduction, thus indicating the high toxicity potential of photo-transformation products of diclofenac at concentration levels that may come close to environmental concentrations of residual diclofenac after degradation (Schmitt-Jansen et al., 2007).

CONCLUSION

Diclofenac was reported to have caused poisoning of three species of vultures on Indian subcontinent (*Gyps bengalensis*, *Gyps indicus*, and *Gyps tenuirostris*), and causing their decline in population by 97% (Sumpter, 2010). As a result, an increasing body of research has investigated the ecotoxicological effects of diclofenac on non-target organisms, and has mainly focused on acute effects on aquatic organisms. The study by Memmert et al., (2013), concluded that it was the findings of chronic toxicity and bioconcentration in fish that are currently the main basis for many stakeholders to conclude that even the low concentrations of diclofenac measured in surface waters present a high risk to the environment. Hence, robust environmental risk assessment, require high quality ecotoxicological data from long-term exposure studies on diclofenac. Therefore, more studies need to be done on the chronic effect of diclofenac based on the low concentrations that are detected in the environment. Chronic toxicity should inform future directive and policy on control of diclofenac. There is need to prevent and to reduce diclofenac levels as a pollutant in the environment. Since there is no information of biotransformation products that are associated with diclofenac in the environment, it's difficult to predict the effects of such compounds to organisms. Pharmaceuticals are intrinsically bioactive compounds that are able to cause potential damage on living systems, target and non-target organisms. The damage can be caused through synergistic or antagonistic effects which may not only be as a result of the diclofenac molecule but its metabolites and products of their reaction with other environmental molecules present. In addition the ability of diclofenac and its metabolites to change and to accumulate in the environment should be realized (Baranauskaitė and Dvarionienė, 2014). If policy and control on proper management of pharmaceutical active ingredients disposal and remediation from the environment is not enforced, these compound concentrations are projected to increase in the environment. Example, the report from the study by Johnson et al., (2014) estimated that over 2% by length of rivers would reach concentrations greater than the proposed EQS of for fresh water of 100 ngL^{-1} for diclofenac (EQS for Saltwater 0.01 μgL^{-1}). Hence, there is a need for high quality ecotoxicological data from long-term exposure studies with diclofenac to allow for a robust environmental risk assessment.

REFERENCES

ACS Daten Bank. Diclofenac. Organic carbon – water partition coefficient (K_{OC}). 2004.

Andreozzi, R.; Marotta, R.; Nicklas. P. Pharmaceuticals in STP effluents and their solar photodegradation in aquatic environment. *Chemosphere.* 2003; 50, 1319 – 1330.

Avdeef, A.; Box, K. J.; Comer, J. E. A.; Hibbert, C.; Tam, K. Y. pH-metric logP 10. Determination of liposomal membrane-water partition coefficients of ionizable drugs. *Pharmaceut Res.* 1998; 15, 209 - 215.

Baranauskaitė, I.; Dvarionienė, J. Presence and Detection of Pharmaceutical Substances (Diclofenac, 17-β-estradiol, 17-α-etilinestradiol) in the Environment. Future Challenges for Lithuania. *Environmental Research, Engineering and Management.* 2014; No. 2, (68), P. 25 – 40.

Benotti, M. J.; Trenholm, R. A.; Vanderford, B. J.; Holady, J. C.; Stanford, B. D.; Snyder, S. A. Pharmaceuticals and endocrine disrupting compounds in U.S. drinking water. *Environmental Science & Technology.* 2009; 43, (3), 597–603.

Bessa, V. S.; Moreira, L. S.; Tiritan,ME..; Castro, P. M. L. (2017). Enrichment of bacterial strains for the biodegradation of diclofenac and carbamazepine from activated sludge. *International Biodeterioration & Biodegradation.* 2017; Volume 120, Pages 135-142.

BIO Intelligence Service. Study on the environmental risks of medicinal products, Final Report prepared for Executive Agency for Health and Consumers. 201). https://ec.europa.eu/health//sites/health/files/files/environment/study_environment.pdf.

Chen, J. B.; Gao, H. W.; Zhang, Y. L.; Zhang, Y.; Zhou, X. F.; Li Ch,Q.; Gao, H. P. Developmental toxicity of diclofenac and elucidation of gene regulation in zebrafish (Danio rerio). *Sci. Rep.* 2014; 4, 4841.

Cuklev, F.; Kristiansson, E.; Fick, J.; Asker, N.; Forlin, L.; Larsson, D. G. J. Diclofenac in fish: blood plasma levels similar to human therapeutic levels affect global hepatic gene expression. *Environ Toxicol Chem.* 2011; 30. (9). 2126-34.

European Chemical Bureau, Institute for Health and Consumer Protection. Technical Guidance Document on Risk Assessment (TGD II), 2008. http://ecb.jrc.it/documents/TECHNICAL_GUIDANCE_DOCUMENT.

European Commission Sub-Group on Review of the Priority Substances List. Diclofenac EQS dossier. 2011. Available online: https://circabc.europa.eu/sd/a/d88900c0-68ef-4d34-8bb1-baa9af220afd/Diclofenac%20EQS%20dossier%202011.pdf.

Fent, K.; Weston, A. A.; Caminada, D. Ecotoxicology of human pharmaceuticals. *Aquatic Toxicol.* 2006; 76, 122 – 159.

Ferrari, B.; Mons, R.; Vollat, B.; Fraysse, B.; Paxéus, N.; Lo Giudice, R.; Pollio, A.; Garric, J. Environmental risk assessment of six human pharmaceuticals: are the current environmental risk assessment procedures sufficient for the protection of the aquatic environment? *Environ Toxicol Chem.* 2004 May; 23, (5), 1344-54.

Gardner, M.; Jones, V.; Comber, S.; Scrimshaw, M. D.; Coello-Garcia, T.; Cartmell, E.; Lester, J.; Ellor, B. Performance of UK wastewater treatment works with respect to trace contaminants. *Sci. Total Environ.* 2013; 456 - 457, 359 - 369.

Groening, J.; Held, C.; Garten, C.; Claussnitzer, U.; Kaschabek, S. R.; Schloemann, M.; Transformation of diclofenac by the indigenous microflora of river sediments and identification of a major intermediate. *Chemosphere*, 2007; 69, 509 - 516.

Guiloski, I. C.; Ribas, J. L. C.; Pereira, L. D. S.; Neves, A. P. P.; Assis, H. C. S. D. Effects of trophic exposure to dexamethasone and diclofenac in freshwater fish. *Ecotoxicol Environ Saf.* 2015; 114, 204-211.

Heberer, T.; Stan, H. J. Determination of clofibric acid and N-(Phenylsulfonyl)-sarcosine in sewage, river and drinking water. *Int. J. Environ. Anal. Chem.*, 1997; 67: 113–124.

Heberer T.; Reddersen K.; Mechlinski A. From municipal sewage to drinking water: Fate and removal of pharmaceutical residues in the aquatic environment in urban areas. *Water Sci Technol.* 2002; 46:81–88.

Isidori, M.; Nardelli, A.; Parrella, A.; Pascarella, L.; Previtera, L. A multispecies study to assess the toxic and genotoxic effect of pharmaceuticals: furosemide and its photoproduct. *Chemosphere.* 2006; 63, 785 – 793.

Jjemba, P. K. Technologies for removing PPCPs. In: Jjemba P. K. (Editor). *Pharma-ecology: The Ocurrence and Fate of Pharmaceuticals and Personal Care Products in the Environment.* New Jersey: John Wiley & Sons. 2008; Chapter 5.

Johnson, A. C.; Dumont, E.; Williams, R. J.; Oldenkamp, R.; Cisowska, I.; Sumpter, J. P. Do concentrations of ethinylestradiol, estradiol, and diclofenac in European rivers exceed proposed EU environmental quality standards? *Environ. Sci. Technol.* 2013; 47, (21), 1229 7-12304.

Karlsson, M. V.; Marshall, S.; Gouin, T.; Boxall, AB. Routes of uptake of diclofenac, fluoxetine, and triclosan into sediment-dwelling worms. *Environ Toxicol Chem.* 2016; 35(4), 836-42. doi: 10.1002/etc.3020.

Kimosop, S. J.; Getenga, Z. M.; Orata, F.; Okello, V. A.; Cheruiyot, J K. Residue levels and discharge loads of antibiotics in wastewater treatment plants (WWTPs), hospital lagoons, and rivers within Lake Victoria Basin, Kenya. *Environmental Monitoring and Assessment.* 2016; 188:532.

Kimura, K.; Hara, H.; Watanabe, Y. Elimination of selected acidic pharmaceuticals from municipal wastewater by an activated sludge system and membrane bioreactors. *Environ. Sci. Technol.* 2007; 41, (10), 3708 - 3714.

KNAPPE. Knowledge and Need Assessment on Pharmaceutical Products in Environmental Waters; Sixth Framework Programme, Report on environmental impact and health effects of PPs, 2007.

Kümmerer, K. Pharmaceuticals in the Environment: Sources, Fate, Effects and Risks, third ed. *Springer*, Berlin, Heidelberg. 2008.

Langenhoff, A.; Inderfurth, N.; Veuskens, T.; Schraa, G.; Blokland, M.; Kujawa-Roeleveldk. Rijnaarts, H. Microbial removal of the pharmaceutical compounds ibuprofen and diclofenac from wastewater. *BioMed Res. Int. Article.* 2013; ID 325806, 9 pages.

Lee, J.; Ji, K.; Kho, Y. L.; Kim, P.; Choi, K. Chronic exposure to diclofenac on two freshwater cladocerans and Japanese medaka. *Ecotoxicol Environ Saf.* 2011; 74, 1216 - 1225.

LUBW, 2014. Landesanstalt für Umwelt, Messungen und Naturschutz Baden-Württemberg, Spurenstoffinventar der Fließgewässer in Baden-Württemberg [*State Institute for the Environment, Measurements and Nature Conservation Baden-Württemberg, trace substances inventory of the rivers in Baden-Württemberg*] Results from the analyses of waste water treatment plants in 2012/2013.

Memmert U.; Peither A.; Burri R.; Weber K.; Schmidt T.; Sumpter J. P.; Hartmann A. Diclofenac: new data on chronic Toxicity and bioconcentration in fish. *Environ. Toxicol. Chem.* 2013; 32, 442.

Memmert, U.; Peither, A.; Roland Burri, R.; Weber, K.; Schmidt, T.; John, P.; Sumpter, J. P. Hartmann, A. (2013) Diclofenac: New data on chronic toxicity and bioconcentration in fish. *Environmental Toxicology and Chemistry.* 32, (2), 442-52.

Oaks, J. L.; Gilbert, M.; Virani, M. Z.; Watson, R. T.; Meteyer, C. U.; Rideout, B. A.; Shivaprasad, H. L.; Ahmed, S.; Chaudry, M. J. I.; Arshad, M.; Mahmood, S.; Ali, A.; Khan, A. A. (2004) Diclofenac residues as the cause of population decline of vultures in Pakistan. *Nature*, 2004; 427, 630 - 633.

Oaks, J. L.; Watson, R. T. South Asian vultures in crisis: Environmental contamination with a pharmaceutical. In: Elliott JE, Bishop CA, Morrissey CA, editors. Wildlife ecotoxicology forensic approaches. New York (NY): *Springer.* 2011; p 413 – 441.

Packer, J. L.; Werner, J. J.; Latch, D. E.; McNeill, K.; Arnold, W. A, Photochemical fate of pharmaceuticals in the environment: naproxen, diclofenac, clofibric acid, and ibuprofen. *Aquat Sci.* 2003; 65, 342–351.

Perez-Estrada, L. A.; Malato, S.; Gernjak, W.; Agueram, A.; Thurman, E. M.; Ferrer, I.; Photo-Fenton Degradation of Diclofenac: Identification of Main Intermediates and Degradation Pathway. *Environ. Sci. Technol.*, 2005; 39, (21), pp 8300 – 8306.

Prakash, V.; Pain, D. J.; Cunningham, A. A.; Donald, P. F.; Prakash, N.; Verma, A.; Gargi, R.; Sivakumar, S.; Rahmani, A. R. (2003) Catastrophic collapse of Indian white-backed Gyps bengalensis and long-billed Gyps indicus vulture populations. *Biological Conservation*, 2003; 109, 381 - 390.

Praskova, E.; Plhalova, L.; Chromcova, L.; Stepanova, S.; Bedanova, I.; Blahova, J.; Hostovsky, M.; Skoric, M.; Maršálek, P.; Voslarova, E.; Svobodova, Z. Effects of Subchronic Exposure of Diclofenac on Growth, Histopathological Changes, and Oxidative Stress in Zebrafish (Danio rerio). *Scientific World Journal*. 2014; 5, 2014:645737. doi: 10.1155/2014/645737.

Santos, L. H. M. L. M.; Araújo A. N.; Fachini A.; Pena A.; Delerue-Matos C.; Montenegro M. C. B. S. M,. 2010. Ecotoxicological aspects related to the presence of pharmaceuticals in the aquatic environment. *Journal of Hazardous Materials*, 2010; Vol. 175, pp. 45- 95.

Sari S.; Ozdemir G.; Yangin-Gomec C.; Zengin G. E.; Topuz E.; Aydin E., et al., "Seasonal variation of diclofenac concentration and its relation with wastewater characteristics at two municipal wastewater treatment plants in Turkey," *Journal of Hazardous Materials*, 2014; vol. 272, pp. 155-164,

Scheytt, T.; Mersmann, P.; Lindstädt, R.; Hebere, T. Determination of sorption coefficients of pharmaceutically active substances carbamazeping, diclofenac, and ibuprofen, in sandy sediments. *Chemosphere*. 2005; 60: 245-253.

Schmitt-Jansen, M.; Bartels, P.; Adler, N.; Altenburger, R. Phytotoxicity assessment of diclofenac and its phototransformation products. *Anal Bioanal Chem*. 2007; 387, 1389-1396. doi:10.1007/s00216-006-0825-3.

Schwaiger, J.; Ferling, H.; Mallow, U.; Wintermayr, H.; Negele, D. R. Toxic effectsofthenon-steroidalanti-inflammatorydrugdiclofenac Part I: Histopathological alterations and bioaccumulation in rainbow trout. *Aquat Toxicol*. 2004; 68, 141 - 150.

Stan, H. J.; Heberer T. Pharmaceuticals in the aquatic environment. *Water Anal*. 1997; 25, 20–23.

Sumpter, J. P. Pharmaceuticals in the Environment: Moving from Problem to a Solution. In: Kümerer K. and Hempel M. (Editors). *Green and*

Sustainable Pharmacy. Heidelberg, Germany: *Springer-Verlag. 2010;* Chapter 2.

Syracuse Science Center. Database of experimental octanol-water partition coefficients (LogP). - Homepage http://esc-plaza.s yrres.com/ interkow/kowdemo.htm. 2002.

Ter Laak, TL. Van der Aa, M.; Houtman, CJ; Stoks, PC; Van Wezel, AP.; Relating environmental concentrations of pharmaceuticals to consumption: a mass balance approach for the river Rhine. *Environ Int.* 2010; 36: 403.

Ternes, T. A.; Joss, A.; Siegrist. Scrutinizing pharmaceuticals and personal care products in wastewater treatment. *Environmental Science and Technology*, 2004; 38(20), 392A-399A. http://doi.org/10.1021/es040 639t.

Ternes, T. A. Analytical methods for the determination of pharmaceuticals in aqueous environmental samples. *Trends Anal Chem* 2001; 20:419 - 434.

Vazquez-Roig, P.; Segarra, R.; Blasco, C.; Andreu, V.; Picó, Y. Determination of pharmaceuticals in soils and sediments by pressurized liquid extraction and liquid chromatography tandem mass spectrometry. *J Chromatogr A.* 2010; 16:1217(16), 2471-83.

Vieno, N.; Sillanpää, M. Fate of diclofenac in municipal wastewater treatment plant - A review. *Environment International.* 2014. Volume 69, August 2014, Pages 28-39.

Vulliet E., Cren-Olive C., Grenier-Loustalot M. F. Occurrence of pharmaceuticals and hormones in drinking water treated from surface waters. *Environmental Chemistry Letters.* 2011; 9:103–114.

Weber, F. A.; aus der Beek, T.; Bergmann, A.; Carius, A.; Grüttner, G.; Hickmann, S.; Ebert, I.; Hein, A.; Küster, A.; Rose, J.; Koch-Jugl, J.; Stolzenberg, H. C. *Pharmaceuticals in the environment – the global perspective Occurrence, effects, and potential cooperative action under SAICM.* German Federal Environmental Agency (UBA). 2014. Available at: https://www.umweltbundesamt.de/en/database-pharmaceuticals-in-the-environment-0.

Weigel, S.; Kuhlmann, J., Hühnerfuss, H. Drugs and personal care products as ubiquitous Pollutants: occurrence and distribution of clofibric acid, caffeine and DEET in the North Sea. *Sci. Total Environ.* 2002; 295:131-141.

Zhang, Y.; Geißen, S. U.; Gal, C. Carbamazepine and diclofenac: Removal in wastewater treatment plants and occurrence in water bodies. *Chemosphere.* 2008; 73, 1151–1161.

Zhang, Y.; Kong, H.; Fang, Y.; Nishinari, K.; Phillips, G. O. Schizophyllan: a review of its structure, properties, bioactivity and recent developments. *Bioactive Carbohydr. Dietary Fibre* 1. 2013; 53–71. 10.1016/j.bcdf.2013.01.002.

Zhaoqi, J.; Tao L.; Hong. T. Electrochemical degradation of diclofenac for pharmaceutical wastewater treatment. *Int. J. Electrochem. Sci.* 2017; 127807–7816.

In: Environmental Pharmacology of Diclofenac ISBN: 978-1-53617-466-3
Editor: Eugenia Yiannakopoulou © 2020 Nova Science Publishers, Inc.

Chapter 4

SOURCE OF DICLOFENAC IN DRINKING AND WASTEWATER

Noshin Hashim[1,], Aveen Alkhatib[2] and Ajay K. Ray[1]*
[1]Faculty of Engineering, Western University, London Ontario Canada
[2]Bayer Crop Science, West Sacramento, California US

ABSTRACT

Water pollution has become an increasing problem due to population growth, industrialization, urbanization and shifting climate patterns and it's increasing the demand for potable water. Pharmaceutical compounds, personal care products and endocrine disrupting compounds make up a substantial portion of water pollution. One of the commonly and heavily used pharmaceutical active ingredients is Diclofenac (DCF). Both DCF and its byproducts were found to possess a bio-accumulative risk due to its steady input into recipient waters and found to have toxic effects on cell function of aquatic animals. The problem aggregated due to the unreliability of the available conventional water treatment methods. As a

---

[*] Corresponding Author's Email: nhashim@uwo.ca.; Noshin Hashim PhD, Lecturer, Faculty of Engineering, Western University, London Ontario Canada.

result, Advanced Oxidation Processes (AOPs) has emerged to address this issues. Photocatalysis is a unique growing AOP for water treatment process that can be an alternative and effective solution for DCF treatment found in water sources. In this chapter, the source of DCF and its toxic byproducts in water sources are explained. Treatment options for removal of DCF and other pharmaceutical contaminants are introduced. In addition, the mechanism of photocatalysis, in treating water pollution such as DCF is described.

Keywords: diclofenac, DCF, advanced oxidation processes, AOP, toxic, photocatalysis

NOMENCLATURE

AOPs	Advanced oxidation processes
DCF	Diclofenac, a model compound for this kinetic study
EC_{50}	Median Effective Concentration (required to induce a 50% effect)
EDCs	Endocrine Disrupting Compounds
e^-	Electron
h^+	Hole
NSAIDS	No-steroidal anti-inflammatory drugs
PCP_s	Pharmaceutical and personal care products
WWTP	Wastewater treatment plant
h	Plank's constant ($\sim 6.6 \times 10^{-34}$ J.s)
c	Speed of light (3.0×10^8 m/s)

Greek Letters

λ	Wavelength of incident light, nm

1. INTRODUCTION

Water pollution is an increasing problem in a world that faces declining water and energy sources. Despite the fact that over 70% of the earth's surface is covered by water, less than 1% of all freshwater is accessible for human use. Population growth, industrialization, urbanization and shifting climate patterns are increasing the demand for potable water.

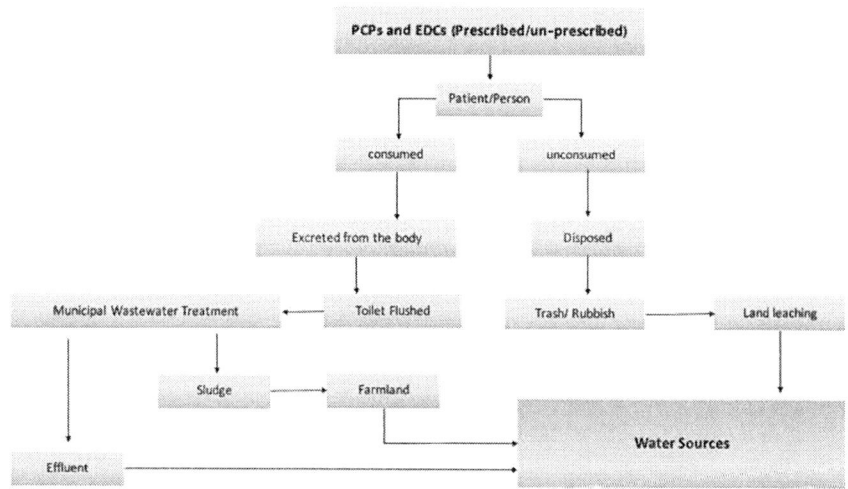

Figure 1. EDCs and PCs pathways to the water sources.

Wastewater reuse and value recovery from wastewater have resulted in market growths for sustainable technologies in water and wastewater treatment. However, water pollution threatens our health and environment and has become an issue of major social and economic concern (Klavarioti et al. 2009; Perazzolo et al. 2010; Miège et al. 2009; Hashim et al. 2017).

Anthropocentric factors are also contributing to pollution in freshwater sources, of which pharmaceuticals and personal care products (PCPs) make up a substantial portion. Water resources are becoming increasingly contaminated with these toxic compounds and it is an immediate and important challenge in a world that faces increasing pollution and decreasing energy resources (Fent et al. 2006; Fent et al. 1996; Hallare, Köhler, and Triebskorn 2004; Stülten et al. 2008; Saravanan et al. 2017; Ziylan et al. 2011a). These emerging contaminants are of increasing concern as a threat to human and aquatic health and are being considered by government regulators around the world (Nahar et al. 2006). The problem aggravates due to the unreliability of conventional treatment methods (Klavarioti, Mantzavinos, and Kassinos 2009) (Figure 1). Extensive use of emerging contaminants including endocrine disrupting compounds (EDCs), PCPs, and pharmaceutically active compounds with mutagenic, genotoxic, and carcinogenic effects are also of increasing prevalence of water resources (Perazzolo et al. 2010; Miège et al. 2009).

1.1. Diclofenac

One of the most commonly detected and heavily used pharmaceuticals is Diclofenac (DCF) [2-(2,6-dichloroaniline) phenylacetic acid]. It is ingested as a pharmaceutical active to reduce inflammation in patients and is one of the most heavily used no-steroidal anti-inflammatory drugs (NSAIDs) around the world. In water sources, the main contamination pathways are identified to be through domestic use. While DCF is found at low concentrations (ng/L and μg/L), it possesses a bio-accumulative risk due to its steady input into recipient waters (Ziylan and Ince 2011a; Agüera et al. 2005; Mehrotra et al. 2003). It has toxic effects on cell function of aquatic animals and is known to be the cause of major vulture population decline in western Asia.[7,15,18] Concentrations as low as ng/l levels were reported to inhibit cell proliferation by affecting their physiology and morphology (Hashim et al. 2017; Fent et al. 2006; Fent 1996).

Recent research reported that sub-chronic exposure to diclofenac at ng/l levels could interfere with the biochemical functions of fish and cause tissue damage as well. DCF also presents the highest acute aquatic toxicity (Fent et al. 1996). Therefore, it increases the potential to harm organisms at a cellular level. The presence of 1 μgL^{-1} of DCF has been reported to damage liver and kidney cell functions in aquatic animals (Hallare et al. 2004)

Furthermore, ingestion of DCF by birds results in death shortly after exposure to the contaminated source (Stülten et al. 2008). The potency or half the maximal effective concentration (EC50) for DCF reported in the literature is considered to be very toxic to bacteria (EC50 < 1mg/L) and algae (EC50 = 1-10mg/L) (Fujishima, Zhang, and Tryk 2007; 2008). It also has the 8th highest average mass load in the secondary effluent of municipal wastewater treatment plants out of 73 reviewed pharmaceuticals (Nahar et al. 2006; Ling et al. 2008). As a result, DCF has been added to the Water Framework Directive watch list of priority substances under the European Union as of 2013. Table 1 summarizes the physical property, chemical and aquatic toxicity of DCF.

Table 1. Chemical, the physical and aquatic toxicity of DCF (Saravanan et al. 2017)

Drug	Molecular Weight (g/mol)	Solubility (mg/L)	pKa (at 20°C)	$EC_{50}(\frac{mg}{L})$	
				daphnia	alage
DCF	296.2	2.37	4.16	22-68	72
Chemical Structure					

Table 2 indicates a relative consumption of DCF around the world. In addition, it shows the country wise occurrence of DCF in surface waters.

DCF elimination is not achieved using conventional wastewater treatment methods, as it can be seen from Table 2 (inlet and outlet stream of wastewater treatment plant (WWTP). This is because the conventional wastewater treatment is based on physical, mechanical, biological and chemical processes (Table 3). The conventional processes are unreliable for completely eliminating the mentioned contaminates because, filtration and adsorption of contaminated from wastewater improve the quality of water to certain extent but, it creates post-process waste. Therefore, causing a new stream of waste that are pollutant rich, and need to be further treated. In addition, some of the pollutants found in water are non-biodegradable, for which a tertiary treatment is required.

The flexibility of the treatment, efficiency, cost-effectiveness and eco-friendliness of a process is essential and therefore, a great amount of research has been contacted to develop such a process (Saravanan et al. 2017). As a result, Advanced Oxidation Processes (AOPs) have emerged to address this issue while complying with environmental regulations.

Table 2. Global consumption rates and country-wise occurrence of DCF

DCF (tons/year)	Location	Surface Concentration (mg/L)	WWTP influent (μg/L)	WWTP effluent (μg/L)	Location
4.5	Switzerland (Fent et al. 2006)	0.001-0.37	0.470-1.9	0.320-0.930	Switzerland (Buser, Poiger, and Müller 1998)
1	Finland (Lindqvist et al. 2005)	1.03	3.02	2.51	Germany (Heberer 2002)
86	Germany (Nikolaou et al. 2007)		0.105-4.11	2.51	France (Miège et al. 2009)
26	England (Jones et al. 2002)		2.59	1.97	South Korea (Henschel et al. 1997)
4.4	Australia (Tambosi et al. 2010)	0.15	3.5	0.81	Germany (Sirbu D., Cadariu and Moldovan 2006)
43	US (Thacker et al. 2005)	0.020-0.150	3.1	1.5	Austria (Sirbu D., Cadariu and Moldovan 2006)
1014	World (Zhang et al. 2008)			0.25-5.45	France, Italy, Sweden (Andreozzi, Marotta, and Paxéus 2003)

An extensive effort has been made by several authors to find effective solutions for elimination of DCF from the water. The type of processes (including the conventional and AOPs) and the effectiveness of each in eliminating DCF from water are listed in Table 3.

2. ADVANCED OXIDATION PROCESS (AOP) AS A TREATMENT METHOD FOR DCF

Filtration technologies, ultraviolet (UV) radiation, and advanced oxidation processes (AOPs) are known methods for removing contaminants in water (Ziylan et al. 2011b) As noted above use of membranes and filters trap contaminants removed from the water, however, the disposal process of these membranes and filters pose risks to the environment (Nahar, Hasegawa, and Kagaya 2006; Ling, Sun, and Zhou 2008). In this regard and AOPs are more reliable in the sense that the contaminants are converted into stable, harmless inorganic compounds such as carbon dioxide, water and mineral salts.

There are several types of AOPs, but they are mostly classified into two sections, *Photochemical AOPs*, and *Non-photochemical AOPs*. From Table 3, ozone/hydroxide ozone/hydrogen peroxide (O_3/H_2O_2), Fenton and photo-Fenton are considered photochemical AOPs. Photochemical AOPs, on the other hand, can be homogenous, meaning both the catalyst and the reactant exist in the same phase (such as UV/H_2O_2), or it can be a heterogeneous process, where catalyst and reactants are in two different phases (UV/TiO_2) (Nahar, Hasegawa, and Kagaya 2006).

2.1. Photocatalysis

Photocatalysis simple means the acceleration of a chemical reaction by light in presence of a catalyst. Photocatalysis is composed of two Greek words, photo (light) and catalysis (catalyst). Therefore, the process requires the energy provided by the light (UV or solar) to speed a chemical reaction that takes place in a system.

There are two types of photocatalysis: *homogenous* and *heterogeneous*. In a homogenous process, both the catalyst and the reactant exist in the same phase. In heterogeneous photocatalysis, the catalyst and reactants are in two different phases. An example of homogenous process and photocatalyst includes ozone and photo-Fenton systems (see Table 3). On the other hand, the most common heterogeneous photocatalyst are transition metal oxides and semiconductors, such as titanium dioxide (TiO_2).

Among the two types, heterogeneous photocatalysis, using a semiconductor catalyst, particularly TiO_2 is an emerging technology (Hoffmann et al. 1995; Ling, Sun, and Zhou 2008; Zhou et al. 2003). This due to photocatalysis treatment presents multiple advantages (Ziylan and Ince 2011a) when compared to conventional methods and these are but not limited to;

- The process can be achieved without any pH adjustments or the use of toxic compounds as it requires only dissolved oxygen (air); (Pérez-Estrada et al. 2005)
- TiO_2 is inexpensive and it is commercially available in various crystalline forms with a wide range of particle characteristics. In addition, it is non-toxic, photochemically stable and can be reused;
- TiO_2 can also be modified to further enhance its photo-catalytic activity;
- A low-energy light source such as the UV-A is sufficient to promote catalyst activation; solar visible, full spectrum and UV-LED light could also be used as alternative sources of energy when the catalyst is suitably modified (Mehrotra et al. 2003; Hashim et al. 2014; Chowdhury et al. 2012).

In short, photocatalytic treatment can be defined as the conversion of an organic pollutant from water (or air) sources to carbon dioxide (CO_2), water (H_2O), and mineral acid by means of light (photon) activated catalyst.

2.2.1. Semiconductor Photocatalyst

A photocatalytic reaction needs sufficient energy (UV, or visible light), and a photocatalyst. A great number of semiconductors (Table 4) are utilized as a photocatalyst. The energy requirement for activation of a semiconductor depends on its characteristics. The minimum energy (light) wavelength (λ_{min}) required to photoexcite catalysts depends on its bandgap energy.

Table 3. Most common AOPs for water and wastewater treatment

Treatment Processes	References	Removal Rate %
Conventional Method		
Settling	Tanaka et al. (Kim and Tanaka 2009)	-
Coagulation		
(a) Fe$_2$(SO$_4$)$_3$	Tuhkanen et al. (N Vieno, Tuhkanen, and Kronberg 2006)	66
(b) Al$_2$(SO$_4$)$_3$	Tuhkanen et al. (Lindqvist, Tuhkanen, and Kronberg 2005)	-
Sand filtration	Vieno et al. (N Vieno, Tuhkanen, and Kronberg 2006)	10
Activated carbon	Vieno et al. (Niina Vieno and Sillanpää 2014) Westeroff et al. (Westerhoff et al. 2005)	39
Disinfection		
(a) Cl$_2$ (up to 3.8 mg/L)	Benotti et al. (Benotti and Snyder 2009) Vieno et al. (Nina Vieno 2007)	80-95
(b) O$_3$ (up to 1.5 mg/L)	Ternes et al. (Ternes et al. 2002)	More than 99
AOPs		
Photolysis		
(a) Solar light	Tanaka et al. (Kim and Tanaka 2009)/Canonica et al. (Canonica, Meunier, and von Gunten 2008)	4
(b) UV light	Tanaka et al. (Kim, Yamashita, and Tanaka 2009)/Canonica et al. (Canonica, Meunier, and von Gunten 2008)	90-100
(c) UV light/H$_2$O$_2$	Yamashita et al. (Kim, Yamashita, and Tanaka 2009)	More than 90
Photocatalysis		
(a) TiO$_2$/UV light	Pérez-Estrada et al. (Pérez-Estrada et al. 2005)	100
(b) TiO$_2$-Dye/Solar light	Hashim et al. (Hashim, Natarajan, and Ray 2014; Hashim et al. 2017)	100
Fenton		
(a) TiO$_2$/UV light	Pérez-Estrada et al. (Pérez-Estrada et al. 2005)	100
(b) Sonocatalysis	Naddeo et al. (Naddeo et al. 2009)	35

Among semiconductor photocatalyst, TiO$_2$ has shown excellent results based on the literature studies (Perazzolo et al. 2010; Qi et al. 2013; Michael et al. 2010). It is a very well known and most utilized semiconductor studied around the globe because of its multidisciplinary nature. The diverse application of this material, and the principle of photocatalytic process taking place on the surface of TiO$_2$ make it applicable to a wide range of technologies such a water purification for degradation of organic and inorganic pollutants in water bodies, such as for self-cleaning surfaces; materials coated on the surface of window blinds, titles, kitchen or bathroom (Chowdhury et al. 2012; Zhang et al. 2006; Fujishima et al. 2007; 2008; Diebold et al. 2003)

TiO_2 is cheap and is commercially available in various crystalline forms with a wide range of particle characteristics. In addition, TiO_2 is nontoxic and photochemically stable and can be reused for long period of time, and catalyst photo-activation can be achieved with a low-energy UV-A light source (Stülten et al. 2008; Nahar et al. 2006; Ling et al. 2008).

2.2.2. Photocatalytic Mechanism

In order to visualize the following process better, imagine a liter container with high concentration of DCF. To treat this water you decided to utilize an AOP, in this case heterogeneous photocatalysis. You remember that you need a photocatalyst (let's say TiO_2), and energy source (in this case UV light). Therefore, you place a known amount to TiO_2 inside the container, mixing it well, and expose it under a UV lamp. The illumination of a semiconductor or a photocatalyst by light (UV light, $\lambda <$ 380 nm for example) results in the generation of electron/hole (e-/h+) pairs as a primary step in the photo-degradation process (Equation 1 and Figure 2). As a result, oxidation-reduction reactions occur at the photocatalyst surface. The majority of these e-/h+ pairs tend to recombine with the liberation of heat; however, in the presence of dissolved oxygen in a treatment system (assuming the polluted water have enough oxygen), the photo-generated conduction band electrons are trapped, resulting in the formation of a superoxide ion (O_2^-) as shown in Equation 2.

$$Photocatalyst \xrightarrow{\lambda < 380 \text{ nm}} Photocatalyst\ (e^- + h^+) \quad (1)$$

$$O_2 + e^- \rightarrow O_2^- \quad (2)$$

Similarly, the photocatalyst surface-active HO^- group (electron donor), formed by the ionization of water molecule (present in the system) scavenges the valence band holes resulting in the formation of hydroxide radicals (Equations 3 and 4).

$$h^+ + OH^- \rightarrow HO_{ad}^{\cdot} \tag{3}$$

or

$$h^+ + H_2O_{ad} \rightarrow HO_{ad}^{\cdot} + H^+ \tag{4}$$

These reactions moderate the recombination rates and in turn, enhance the photo-degradation rate. The organic molecules (in this case DCF) present in water react with the hydroxyl radicals formed and are eventually oxidized to carbon dioxide, water and mineral acids, as depicted below (Equation 5).

$$Organics + Photocatalyst + h\nu \xrightarrow{HO^{\cdot}} DCF\ (and\ byproducts) \rightarrow$$

$$MineralAcid \rightarrow H_2O + CO_2 \tag{5}$$

2.2. Limitation of Photocatalyst

One of the requirements of the semiconductors (photocatalyst) is the requirement of an artificial UV lamp due to large band gap energy for commonly used photocatalytic materials. Because of the ubiquity of sunlight, the commercial success of this technology depends on the engineering of electronic bands of the photocatalyst for a paradigm-shift to solar-based photocatalysis that could create significant economic and social benefits. As per Planck's law (E = hc/λ), with the use of higher wavelength visible light (λ > 400 nm) as compared to UV (100 < λ (nm) < 400), the energy associated with a larger wavelength light is not sufficient to overcome, for example, TiO_2 band gap (3.2 eV requiring λ < 380 nm). Hence, e−/h+ pairs formation may not take place when sufficient energy is provided.

Table 4. Bandgap energy for various photocatalyst (Wang, Pehkonen, and Ray 2004; Vinu, Akki, and Madras 2010)

Semiconductor (s)	Bandgap (eV)	λ_{min}
TiO_2 (rutile)	3.0	413
TiO_2 (Anatase)	3.2	388
Si	1.1	1127
Fe_2O_3	2.2	564
ZnO	3.2	388
SnO_2	3.5	354
CdS	2.4	517
ZnS	3.7	335

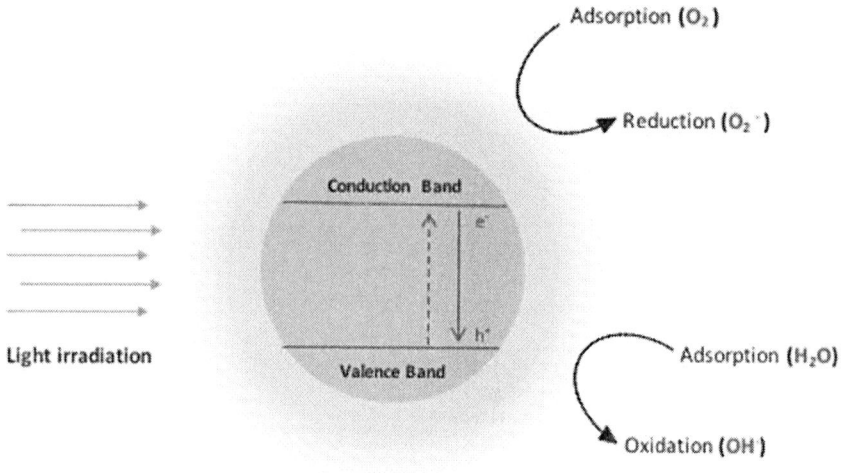

Figure 2. A schematic of the photocatalytic mechanism.

Two approaches address this issue: the first involves reducing the band gap through the addition of *dopants*, thereby allowing light absorption in the visible part of the spectrum (Diebold et al. 2003; Stülten et al. 2008). Dopants can be metal ions (such as CU, Co, Fe and Mn) (Milenova et al. 2014) or nonmetals (such as B, C and S) (In et al. 2007; Ling et al. 2008).

The doping of material into catalyst can enhance it photocatalytic activity and performance. By adding the doping of metals and nonmetals in semiconductors surface we can promote photocatalytic activity in the visible light region.

The second strategy involves *dye-sensitization*. The quintessence of dye-sensitization is the electron injection from the excited dye to the conduction band (CB) of semiconductor (such as TiO_2) and the subsequent interfacial electron transfer. Once the interfacial electron transfer is achieved, the remaining oxidation–reduction steps are the same as before. Hence, the successful synthesis of chemically modified photocatalyst through molecular band engineering will enable sun-powered remediation of environmental pollutants.

In dye sensitization process, the dye molecule is known to adsorb on the semiconductor surface, forming a thin layer of film. This film then adsorbs visible light, and illumination excites the electrons in the dye as a first step; these electrons from the excited dye are then directly injected into the conduction band of the semiconductor, if and only if the energy requirement is met. Figure 3 shows a schematic of the process.

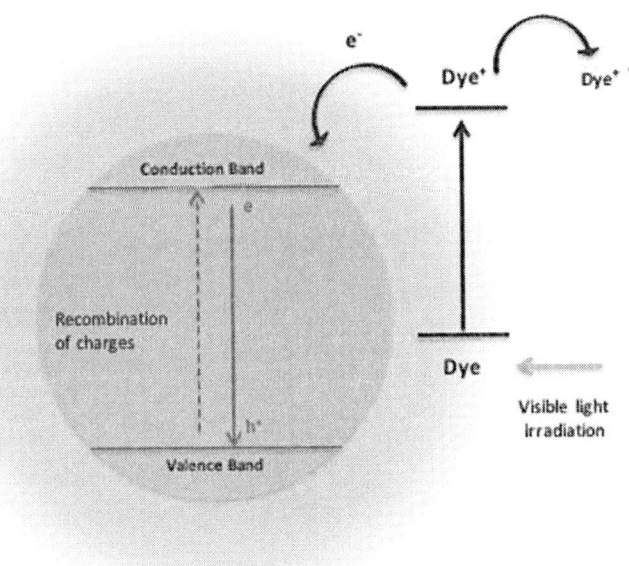

Figure 3. The dye-sensitization mechanism under visible light.

In recent studies, dyes such as acid blue1 (AB1), methylene blue, thionine, eosin Y, rhodamine B, acid red 44, and rhodamine 6G were used to destroy pollutant found in water (Chatterjee et al. 2006; Haque et al. 2007; Qamar et al. 2005; Kojima et al. 2001; Jiang et al. 2008).

Some authors also utilized natural dyes as an alternative source for sensitization (Polo et al. 2004; Wongcharee et al. 2007; Garcia et al. 2003; Polo et al. 2006). These dyes found in plants and fruits are but not limited to mulberry, cabbage, rosella, blue pea, chaste tree fruit, and pomegranate seeds. The efficiency of the process and the rate of degradation are influenced but not limited to the pH of the solution, catalyst loading, and type of semiconductor.

3. DCF Byproducts and Its Toxicity

During the photocatalytic degradation of DCF, new compounds temporally form, known as the intermediates, by-products or transformed compounds (TPs). It is important to study this transformation pathway because the TPs might be more toxic to the environment compared to the model compound. Understanding and analyzing the intermediates is an essential step for their environmental fate.

From the available data in the literature, it can be concluded that the intermediates formed under different AOPs (photolysis, ozonation, sonolysis, heterogeneous photocatalysis, etc.) and conditions result in similar product formation during the photo mineralization of DCF (Coelho et al. 2009; Agüera et al. 2005; Martínez et al. 2011; Calza et al. 2006; Hartmann et al. 2008).

Micheals et al. (Michael et al. 2014). suggest that DCF degradation mainly proceeds by oxidation and hydroxylation reaction between chloroaniline and phenylacetic acid. In addition, the formation of DCF isomers is the result of non-selectivity of hydroxyl radicals (HO·). Thus, confirming a similar reaction mechanism regardless of the type of AOPs utilized to remove DCF from water sources.

Hashim et al. (Hashim et al. 2016) studied the toxicity of untreated and treated DCF (DCF and its by-products) solution was analyzed on *Daphnia Magna* organisms. The rate of mortality of the species was monitored after 24h and 48h exposure times based on the treatment process explained above. The toxicity of treated solution (with intermediate products) was compared to the untreated DCF solution. Figure 4 shows that the untreated DCF solution was less toxic to the organisms compared to the treated solutions. The untreated DCF solution showed an 11% mortality rate of *D. Magna* during the first 24 hours of exposure, which increased to nearly 25% after 48 hours. The mortality rate of the solution of DCF that was irradiated for 15 min showed a much higher mortality rate, nearly 72% in 24h and up to 96% at 48h indicating that the treated DCF, which included the newly formed by-products were much more toxic.

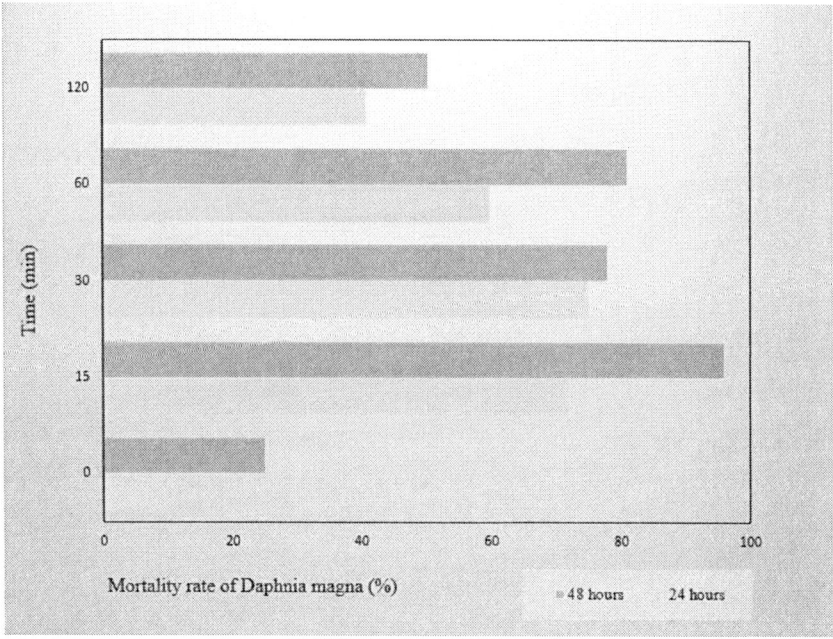

Figure 4. Morality rate of D. Magna after 24 and 48 hours of exposure to untreated and treated solution of DCF. Experimental conditions: Q = 1.15 x 10^{-5} m^3/s, V_L = 4 x 10^{-4} m^3, pH = neutral; T = 298K, O_2 saturated, [EY-TiO$_2$] = 2mg/L, TiO$_2$ = 85 mg/L, solar light intensity = 750W, and [DCF] = 30 mg/L.

Treated DCF solution can be much more toxic than the original untreated DCF solution because photodegradation of DCF contributes to the formation of chloro-derivatives, (Soufan et al. 2012; El Najjar et al. 2013; Qi et al. 2013) this can be observed in Figure 4. As the intermediates formed during the photo mineralization, the higher the toxicity of DCF which was shown to decrease as the degradation process continued. Another reason why the treated solution of DCF is more toxic is due to synergistic effects among the intermediates formed. Michaels et al. and others (Michael et al. 2014; Hapeshi et al. 2010; Michael et al. 2010) studied the effects amongst the transformed by-products and they concluded that the high rate of toxicity is a result of individual and synergistic toxic effects of the DCF and its intermediates.

The toxicity (and formed intermediate products) of the DCF reduced significantly during the 120 min of the reaction. A complete photo mineralization of 30 mg/L of DCF (and intermediate products) using EY-sensitized TiO_2 activated using solar visible was achievable in about 300 minutes.

CONCLUSION

Water pollution is an increasing problem. Population growth, industrialization, urbanization and shifting climate patterns are increasing the demand for potable water. Anthropocentric factors are greatly contributing to pollution in freshwater sources, of which PCPs make up a substantial portion. The water pollution issue also aggravates due to the unreliability of conventional treatment methods.

DCF is one of the most commonly detected and heavily used pharmaceutical active ingredient. Despite the fact that DCF is found at low concentrations (ng/L and μg/L), it still possesses a bio-accumulative risk due to its steady input into recipient waters. It also has toxic effects on cell function of aquatic animals. Based on literature studies and this study, DCF presents the highest acute aquatic toxicity. Therefore, it has the potential to harm organisms at a cellular level.

Treatment processes for DCF from wastewater streams have been reported. Heterogeneous photocatalysis, utilizing TiO_2 as a photocatalyst can be an alternative green solution for water and wastewater treatment. However, the limitation with using TiO_2 as a photocatalyst is the wide band gap energy requirement. This means only about 4% of solar spectrum could be used as a source of energy for any application, making a challenge in industrial application. There is two approaches address this issue: the first involves reducing the band gap through the addition of dopants, thereby allowing light absorption in the visible part of the spectrum. The second strategy involves dye-sensitization of TiO_2 or another photocatalyst. In the literature, however, dye-sensitized TiO_2 was proven to be more efficient by facilitating considerably high DCF degradation rates at visible wavelength compared to TiO_2 photocatalyst under UV light.

Toxicity analysis of the treated (DCF and its by-products) and untreated samples of DCF were also assessed by researchers (Hashim et al. 2016). The treated samples indicated an increase in toxic effect to D. Magna compared to the untreated DCF solution, indicating the formation of harmful by-products. The treated DCF solution can be much more toxic because photodegradation of DCF contributes to the formation of chloro-derivatives. In addition, a synergistic effect among the DCF intermediates formed during the process also contributes to the increase in toxicity.

REFERENCES

Agüera, A., Perez Estrada, L. A., Ferrer, I., Thurman, E. M., Malato, S. & Fernandez-Alba, A. R. (2005). "Application of Time-of-Flight Mass Spectrometry to the Analysis of Phototransformation Products of Diclofenac in Water under Natural Sunlight." *Journal of Mass Spectrometry*, *40* (7), 908–15.

Andreozzi, Roberto., Raffaele, Marotta. & Nicklas, Paxéus. (2003). "Pharmaceuticals in STP Effluents and Their Solar Photodegradation in Aquatic Environment." *Chemosphere*, *50* (10), 1319–30.

Benotti, Mark. & Shane, Snyder. (2009). "Implications for Ground Water Replenishment With." *Ground Water, 47* (4), 499–502.

Buser, Hans Rudolf., Thomas, Poiger. & Markus, D. Müller. (1998). "Occurrence and Fate of the Pharmaceutical Drug Diclofenac in Surface Waters: Rapid Photodegradation in a Lake." *Environmental Science and Technology, 32* (22), 3449–56.

Calza, P., Sakkas, V. a., Medana, C., Baiocchi, C., Dimou, a., Pelizzetti, E. & Albanis, T. (2006). "Photocatalytic Degradation Study of Diclofenac over Aqueous TiO2 Suspensions." *Applied Catalysis B: Environmental, 67* (3–4), 197–205.

Canonica, Silvio., Laurence, Meunier. & Urs, von Gunten. (2008). "Phototransformation of Selected Pharmaceuticals during UV Treatment of Drinking Water." *Water Research, 42* (1–2), 121–28.

Chatterjee, Debabrata., Shimanti, Dasgupta. & Nageswar, N. Rao. (2006). "Visible Light Assisted Photodegradation of Halocarbons on the Dye Modified TiO2 Surface Using Visible Light." *Solar Energy Materials and Solar Cells, 90* (7–8), 1013–20.

Coelho, Alessandra D., Carmen, Sans., Ana, Agera., Maria, Jose Gomez., Santiago, Esplugas. & Marcia, Dezotti. (2009). "Effects of Ozone Pre-Treatment on Diclofenac: Intermediates, Biodegradability and Toxicity Assessment." *Science of the Total Environment, 407* (11), 3572–78.

Diebold, Ulrike. (2003). "The Surface Science of Titanium Dioxide." *Surface Science Reports, 48* (5–8), 53–229.

Fent, K. (1996). "Ecotoxicology of Organotin Compounds." *Critical Reviews in Toxicology, 26* (1), 1–117.

Fent, K., Weston, A. & Caminada, D. (2006). "Ecotoxicology of Human Pharmaceuticals." *Aquatic Toxicology, 76* (2), 122–59.

Fent, K., Weston, A. & Caminda, D. (2006). "Ecotoxicology of Human Pharmaceuticals." *Aquatic Toxicology, 76* (2), 122–59.

Fujishima, Akira., Xintong, Zhang. & Donald, A. Tryk. (2007). "Heterogeneous Photocatalysis: From Water Photolysis to Applications in Environmental Cleanup." *International Journal of Hydrogen Energy, 32* (14), 2664–72.

Fujishima, Akira., Xintong, Zhang. & Donald, A. Tryk. (2008). "TiO2 Photocatalysis and Related Surface Phenomena." *Surface Science Reports, 63* (12), 515–82.

Garcia, Christian Graziani., André, Sarto Polo. & Neyde, Yukie Murakami Iha. (2003). "Fruit Extracts and Ruthenium Polypyridinic Dyes for Sensitization of TiO2 in Photoelectrochemical Solar Cells." *Journal of Photochemistry and Photobiology A: Chemistry, 160* (1–2), 87–91.

Hallare, A. V., Köhler, H. R. & Triebskorn, R. (2004). "Developmental Toxicity and Stress Protein Responses in Zebrafish Embryos after Exposure to Diclofenac and Its Solvent, DMSO." *Chemosphere, 56* (7), 659–66.

Hapeshi, E., Achilleos, a., Vasquez, M. I., Michael, C., Xekoukoulotakis, N. P., Mantzavinos, D. & Kassinos, D. (2010). "Drugs Degrading Photocatalytically: Kinetics and Mechanisms of Ofloxacin and Atenolol Removal on Titania Suspensions." *Water Research, 44* (6), 1737–46.

Haque, M. M. & Muneer, M. (2007). "TiO2-Mediated Photocatalytic Degradation of a Textile Dye Derivative, Bromothymol Blue, in Aqueous Suspensions." *Dyes and Pigments, 75* (2), 443–48.

Hartmann, J., Bartels, P., Mau, U., Witter, M., Tümpling, W. v., Hofmann, J. & Nietzschmann, E. (2008). "Degradation of the Drug Diclofenac in Water by Sonolysis in Presence of Catalysts." *Chemosphere, 70* (3), 453–61.

Hashim, Noshin. (2016). *"Visible Light Driven Photocatalysis for Degradation of Diclofenac,"* Doctoral Tesis.

Hashim, Noshin., Pavithra, Natarajan. & Ajay, K Ray. (2014). "Intrinsic Kinetic Study for Photocatalytic Degradation of Diclofenac under UV and Visible Light." *Industrial and Engineering Chemistry Research*, 53(49), 18637-18646.

Hashim, Noshin., Pavithra, Natarajan. & Ajay, K Ray. (2014). "Intrinsic Kinetic Study for Photocatalytic Degradation of Diclofenac under UV and Visible Light." *Industrial and Engineering Chemistry Research*, 53(49), 18637-18646.

Hashim, Noshin., Shaila, Thakur., Mouska, Patang., Ferdinando, Crapulli. & Ajay, K. Ray. (2017). "Solar Degradation of Diclofenac Using Eosin-Y-Activated TiO2: Cost Estimation, Process Optimization and Parameter Interaction Study." *Environmental Technology (United Kingdom)*, *38* (8), 933–44.

Hashim, Noshin., Shaila, Thakur., Mouska, Patang., Ferdinando, Crapulli. & Ajay, K. Ray. (2017). "Solar Degradation of Diclofenac Using Eosin-Y-Activated TiO2: Cost Estimation, Process Optimization and Parameter Interaction Study." *Environmental Technology (United Kingdom)*, *38* (8), 933–44.

Heberer, T. (2002). "Occurrence, Fate, and Removal of Pharmaceutical Residues in the Aquatic Environment: A Review of Recent Research Data." *Toxicology Letters*, *131*, 5–17.

Henschel, K. P., Wenzel, a., Diedrich, M. & Fliedner, a. (1997). "Environmental Hazard Assessment of Pharmaceuticals." *Regulatory Toxicology and Pharmacology*, *25* (3), 220–25.

Hoffmann, Michael R., Scot, T. Martin., Wonyong, Choi. & Detlef, W. Bahnemannt. (1995). "Environmental Applications of Semiconductor Photocatalysis." *Chemical Reviews*, *95* (1), 69–96.

In, Suil., Alexander, Orlov., Regina, Berg., Felipe, García., Sergio, Pedrosa-Jimenez., Mintcho, S. Tikhov., Dominic, S. Wright. & Richard, M. Lambert. (2007). "Effective Visible Light-Activated B-Doped and B,N-Codoped TiO2photocatalysts." *Journal of the American Chemical Society*, *129* (45), 13790–91.

Jiang, Dong., Yao, Xu., Dong, Wu. & Yuhan, Sun. (2008). "Visible-Light Responsive Dye-Modified TiO2 Photocatalyst." *Journal of Solid State Chemistry*, *181* (3), 593–602.

Jones, O. A. H., Voulvoulis, N. & Lester, J. N. (2002). "Aquatic Environmental Assessment of the Top 25 English Prescription Pharmaceuticals." *Water Research*, *36* (20), 5013–22.

Kim, Ilho. & Hiroaki, Tanaka. (2009). "Photodegradation Characteristics of PPCPs in Water with UV Treatment." *Environment International*, *35* (5), 793–802.

Kim, Ilho., Naoyuki, Yamashita. & Hiroaki, Tanaka. (2009). "Performance of UV and UV/H2O2 Processes for the Removal of Pharmaceuticals Detected in Secondary Effluent of a Sewage Treatment Plant in Japan." *Journal of Hazardous Materials*, *166* (2–3), 1134–40.

Klavarioti, Maria., Dionissios, Mantzavinos. & Despo, Kassinos. (2009). "Removal of Residual Pharmaceuticals from Aqueous Systems by Advanced Oxidation Processes." *Environment International*, *35* (2), 402–17.

Kojima, M., Takahashi, K. & Nakamura, K. (2001). "Cationic Dye-Sensitized Degradation of Sodium Hyaluronate through Photoinduced Electron Transfer in the Upper Excited State." *Photochemistry and Photobiology*, *74* (3), 369–77.

Lindqvist, Nina., Tuula, Tuhkanen. & Leif, Kronberg. (2005). "Occurrence of Acidic Pharmaceuticals in Raw and Treated Sewages and in Receiving Waters." *Water Research*, *39* (11), 2219–28.

Ling, Qincai., Jianzhong, Sun. & Qiyun, Zhou. (2008). "Preparation and Characterization of Visible-Light-Driven Titania Photocatalyst Co-Doped with Boron and Nitrogen." *Applied Surface Science*, *254* (10), 3236–41.

Martínez, C., Canle, M. L., Fernández, M. I., Santaballa J. A. & Faria, J. (2011). "Aqueous Degradation of Diclofenac by Heterogeneous Photocatalysis Using Nanostructured Materials." *Applied Catalysis B: Environmental*, *107* (1–2), 110–18.

Mehrotra, Kanheya., Gregory, S. Yablonsky. & Ajay, K. Ray. (2003). "Kinetic Studies of Photocatalytic Degradation in a TiO2 Slurry System: Distinguishing Working Regimes and Determining Rate Dependences." *Industrial & Engineering Chemistry Research*, *42* (11), 2273–81.

Michael, I., Achilleos, A., Lambropoulou, D., Osorio Torrens, V., Perez, S., Petrovic, M., Barcelo, D. & Fatta-Kassinos, D. (2014). "Proposed Transformation Pathway and Evolution Profile of Diclofenac and Ibuprofen Transformation Products during (Sono)Photocatalysis." *Applied Catalysis B: Environmental*, *147*, 1015–27.

Michael, I., Hapeshi, E., Michael, C. & Fatta-Kassinos, D. (2010). "Solar Fenton and Solar TiO2 Catalytic Treatment of Ofloxacin in Secondary Treated Effluents: Evaluation of Operational and Kinetic Parameters." *Water Research*, *44* (18), 5450–62.

Miège, C., Choubert, J. M., Ribeiro, L., Eusèbe, M. & Coquery, M. (2009). "Fate of Pharmaceuticals and Personal Care Products in Wastewater Treatment Plants Conception of a Database and First Results." *Environmental Pollution*, *157* (5), 1721–26.

Miège, C., Choubert, J. M., Ribeiro, L., Eusèbe, M. & Coquery, M. (2009). "Fate of Pharmaceuticals and Personal Care Products in Wastewater Treatment Plants--Conception of a Database and First Results." *Environmental Pollution*, *157* (5), 1721–26.

Milenova, K., Avramova, I., Eliyas, A., Blaskov, V., Stambolova, I. & Nikoleta, Kassabova. (2014). "Application of Activated M/ZnO (M = Mn, Co, Ni, Cu, Ag) in Photocatalytic Degradation of Diazo Textile Coloring Dye." *Environmental Science and Pollution Research*, *21* (21), 12249–56.

Naddeo, Vincenzo., Vincenzo, Belgiorno., Daniele, Ricco. & Despo, Kassinos. (2009). "Degradation of Diclofenac during Sonolysis, Ozonation and Their Simultaneous Application." *Ultrasonics Sonochemistry*, *16* (6), 790–94.

Nahar, Mst Shamsun., Kiyoshi, Hasegawa. & Shigehiro, Kagaya. (2006). "Photocatalytic Degradation of Phenol by Visible Light-Responsive Iron-Doped TiO2 and Spontaneous Sedimentation of the TiO2 Particles." *Chemosphere*, *65* (11), 1976–82.

Najjar, Nasma Hamdi El., Marie, Deborde., Romain, Journel. & Nathalie, Karpel Vel Leitner. (2013). "Aqueous Chlorination of Levofloxacin: Kinetic and Mechanistic Study, Transformation Product Identification and Toxicity." *Water Research*, *47* (1), 121–29.

Nikolaou, Anastasia., Sureyya, Meric. & Despo, Fatta. (2007). "Occurrence Patterns of Pharmaceuticals in Water and Wastewater Environments." *Analytical and Bioanalytical Chemistry*, *387* (4), 1225–34.

Pankaj, Chowdhury. (2012). "*Solar and visible light driven photocatalysis for sacrificial hydrogen generation and water detoxification with chemically modified TiO2.*" Doctoral Tesis.

Perazzolo, Chiara., Barbara, Morasch., Tamar, Kohn., Anoÿ, Smagnet., Denis, Thonney. & Nathalie, Chèvre. (2010). "Occurrence and Fate of Micropollutants in the Vidy Bay of Lake Geneva, Switzerland. Part I: Priority List for Environmental Risk Assessment of Pharmaceuticals." *Environmental Toxicology and Chemistry*, *29* (8), 1649–57.

Pérez-Estrada, Leónidas A., Sixto, Malato., Wolfgang, Gernjak., Ana, Agüera., Michael Thurman, E., Imma, Ferrer. & Amadeo, R. Fernández-Alba. (2005). "Photo-Fenton Degradation of Diclofenac: Identification of Main Intermediates and Degradation Pathway." *Environmental Science and Technology*, *39* (21), 8300–8306.

Pérez-Estrada, Leónidas a., Sixto, Malato., Wolfgang, Gernjak., Ana, Agüera., Michael Thurman, E., Imma, Ferrer. & Amadeo, R. Fernández-Alba. (2005). "Photo-Fenton Degradation of Diclofenac: Identification of Main Intermediates and Degradation Pathway." *Environmental Science and Technology*, *39* (21), 8300–8306.

Polo, André Sarto. & Neyde, Yukie Murakami Iha. (2006). "Blue Sensitizers for Solar Cells: Natural Dyes from Calafate and Jaboticaba." *Solar Energy Materials and Solar Cells*, *90* (13), 1936–44.

Polo, André Sarto., Melina, Kayoko Itokazu. & Neyde, Yukie Murakami Iha. (2004). "Metal Complex Sensitizers in Dye-Sensitized Solar Cells." *Coordination Chemistry Reviews*, *248* (13–14), 1343–61.

Qamar, M., Saquib, M. & Muneer, M. (2005). "Semiconductor-Mediated Photocatalytic Degradation of Anazo Dye, Chrysoidine Y in Aqueous Suspensions." *Desalination*, *171* (2), 185–93.

Qi, Suzhen., Chen, Wang., Xiaofeng, Chen., Zhaohai, Qin., Xuefeng, Li. & Chengju, Wang. (2013). "Toxicity Assessments with Daphnia Magna of Guadipyr, a New Neonicotinoid Insecticide and Studies of Its Effect on Acetylcholinesterase (AChE), Glutathione S-Transferase (GST), Catalase (CAT) and Chitobiase Activities." *Ecotoxicology and Environmental Safety*, *98*, 339–44.

Saravanan, R., Francisco, Gracia. & Stephen, A. (2017). "*Nanocomposites for Visible Light-Induced Photocatalysis,*" Springer, 19–41.

Saravanan, R., Francisco, Gracia. & Stephen, A. (2017). "*Nanocomposites for Visible Light-Induced Photocatalysis,*" Springer Series (Book Chapter) 19–41.

Sirbu, D., Cadariu, Andrei Achimas. & Zaharie, Moldovan. (2006). "Tenth International Water Technology Conference, IWTC10 2006, Alexandria, Egypt 1151." *Water Technology*, 1151–62.

Soufan, M., Deborde, M. & Legube, B. (2012). "Aqueous Chlorination of Diclofenac: Kinetic Study and Transformation Products Identification." *Water Research*, *46* (10), 3377–86.

Stülten, Dele., Marc, Lamshöft., Sebastian, Zühlke. & Michael, Spiteller. (2008). "Isolation and Characterization of a New Human Urinary Metabolite of Diclofenac Applying LC–NMR–MS and High-Resolution Mass Analyses." *Journal of Pharmaceutical and Biomedical Analysis*, *47* (2), 371–76.

Stülten, Dele., Sebastian, Zühlke., Marc, Lamshöft. & Michael, Spiteller. (2008). "Occurrence of Diclofenac and Selected Metabolites in Sewage Effluents." *Science of the Total Environment*, *405* (1–3), 310–16.

Tambosi, José Luiz., Leonardo, Yassuhiro Yamanaka., Humberto, Jorge José., Regina, De Fátima Peralta Muniz Moreira. & Horst, Friedrich Schröder. (2010). "Recent Research Data on the Removal of Pharmaceuticals from Sewage Treatment Plants (STP)." *Quimica Nova*, *33* (2), 411–20.

Ternes, Thomas A., Martin, Meisenheimer., Derek, McDowell., Frank, Sacher., Heinz, Jürgen Brauch., Brigitte, Haist-Gulde., Gudrun, Preuss., Uwe, Wilme. & Ninette, Zulei-Seibert. (2002). "Removal of Pharmaceuticals during Drinking Water Treatment." *Environmental Science and Technology*, *36* (17), 3855–63.

Thacker, Christine E. & Michael, a. Hardman. (2005). "Molecular phylogeny of basal gobioid fishes: Rhyacichthyidae, Odontobutidae, Xenisthmidae, Eleotridae (Teleostei: Perciformes: Gobioidei)." *Molecular Phylogenetics and Evolution*, (37), 858-871.

Vieno, N., Tuhkanen, T. & Kronberg, L (2006). "Removal of Pharmaceuticals in Drinking Water Treatment: Effect of Chemical Coagulation." *Environmental Technology, 27* (2), 183–92.

Vieno, Niina. & Mika, Sillanpää. (2014). "Fate of Diclofenac in Municipal Wastewater Treatment Plant - A Review." *Environment International, 69*, 28–39

Vieno, Nina. (2007). *Occurrence of Pharmaceuticals in Finnish Sewage Treatment Plants, Surface Waters, and Their Elimination in Drinking Water Treatment Processes.* Tesis Doctoral.

Vinu, R., Spurti, U. Akki. & Giridhar, Madras. (2010). "Investigation of Dye Functional Group on the Photocatalytic Degradation of Dyes by Nano-TiO2." *Journal of Hazardous Materials, 176,* (1–3), 765–73.

Wang, Xiaoling., Pehkonen, S. O. & Ajay, K. Ray. (2004). "Removal of Aqueous Cr(VI) by a Combination of Photocatalytic Reduction and Coprecipitation." *Industrial & Engineering Chemistry Research, 43* (7), 1665–72.

Westerhoff, Paul., Yeomin, Yoon., Shane, Snyder. & Eric, Wert. (2005). "Fate of Endocrine-Disruptor, Pharmaceutical, and Personal Care Product Chemicals during Simulated Drinking Water Treatment Processes." *Environmental Science and Technology, 39* (17), 6649–63.

Wongcharee, Khwanchit., Vissanu, Meeyoo. & Sumaeth, Chavadej. (2007). "Dye-Sensitized Solar Cell Using Natural Dyes Extracted from Rosella and Blue Pea Flowers." *Solar Energy Materials and Solar Cells, 91* (7), 566–71.

Zhang, Xintong., Akira, Fujishima., Ming, Jin., Alexei, V Emeline. & Taketoshi, Murakami. (2006). "Double-Layered TiO2-SiO2 Nanostructured Films with Self-Cleaning and Antireflective Properties." *The Journal of Physical Chemistry B, 110* (50), 25142–48.

Zhang, Yongjun., Sven, Uwe Geißen. & Carmen, Gal. (2008). "Carbamazepine and Diclofenac: Removal in Wastewater Treatment Plants and Occurrence in Water Bodies." *Chemosphere,* (73), 1151-1161.

Zhou, Shuhua. & Ajay, K. Ray. (2003). "Kinetic Studies for Photocatalytic Degradation of Eosin B on a Thin Film of Titanium Dioxide." *Industrial & Engineering Chemistry Research*, *42*, 6020–33.

Ziylan, Asu. & Nilsun, H. Ince. (2011a). "The Occurrence and Fate of Anti-Inflammatory and Analgesic Pharmaceuticals in Sewage and Fresh Water: Treatability by Conventional and Non-Conventional Processes." *Journal of Hazardous Materials*, (187), 24-36.

Ziylan, Asu. & Nilsun, H. Ince. (2011b). "The Occurrence and Fate of Anti-Inflammatory and Analgesic Pharmaceuticals in Sewage and Fresh Water: Treatability by Conventional and Non-Conventional Processes." *Journal of Hazardous Materials*, *187* (1–3), 24–36.

In: Environmental Pharmacology of Diclofenac ISBN: 978-1-53617-466-3
Editor: Eugenia Yiannakopoulou © 2020 Nova Science Publishers, Inc.

Chapter 5

FROM ENVIRONMENTAL PHARMACOLOGY OF DICLOFENAC TO HUMAN PHARMACOLOGY OF DICLOFENAC: IMPLICATIONS FOR HUMAN HEALTH

Eugenia Yiannakopoulou[*]
Department of Biomedical Sciences, Faculty of Health Sciences,
University of West Attica, Athens, Greece

ABSTRACT

Nowadays, there is growing concern on the environmental risks of pharmaceuticals. Pharmaceuticals are present in the environment as a consequence of patient use, drug production and formulation, and improper disposal. Pharmaceuticals pose a risk for aquatic organisms as well as for terrestrial environment. Non-steroidal anti-inflammatory drug diclofenac is one of the most commonly prescribed medicines worldwide. Thus, there is growing concern on the potential environmental risks posed

---

[*] Corresponding Author's Email: nyiannak@teiath.gr; nyiannak@uniwa.gr.

by diclofenac. Diclofenac has been included in the watch list of substances in EU that requires its environmental monitoring in the member states. Diclofenac is known to harmfully affect several environmental species already at concentrations of ≤ 1 μg/l. Most importantly, the environmental impact of diclofenac has implications for human health. Diclofenac has been shown to cause dramatic population declines (>99%) in Gyps vulture species in India and Pakistan, resulting in localised extinctions. The vultures suffered from renal failure after feeding on dead cattle that had been treated with diclofenac. The population decline of vultures has huge ecological consequences, as vultures are natural scavengers that eliminate animal carcasses. Unfed animal carcasses pose a threat for human health. Diclofenac has also been recognized as a threat for plants. Environmental toxicity of diclofenac in plants has implications for human health. Potential human exposure to diclofenac and diclofenac metabolites through dietary intake should be taken into account. Diclofenac as well as other medications and personal care products may contaminate food produce via plant uptake, thus constituting a route for human exposure. For example, crops may take up pharmaceuticals and personal care products through their roots. The paradigm of diclofenac highlights the need for novel environmental policies. Current knowledge on the occurrence of diclofenac in the environment should be improved. Diclofenac might pose an environmental risk in freshwater as well as in treated wastewater. Potential harmful effects of diclofenac in the environment should be monitored. The discipline of environmental pharmacology should be included in the academic curriculum of medicine and the other health sciences. A multidisciplinary approach is needed for ensuring the environmental safety of diclofenac as well as of the other pharmaceuticals.

Keywords: diclofenac, environmental pharmacology, human health, clinical implications, eco- pharmacovigilance

1. INTRODUCTION

Human pharmacology investigates health effects of medications. While health effects of medications are important, recently, there is growing concern on the environmental risks of pharmaceuticals [Boxall et al., 2009, Santos et al., 2010). Pharmaceuticals are a potentially potent group of chemical contaminants, because they are designed to have biological effects at low concentrations. Currently, there are a number of uncertainties associated with the environmental risk assessment of pharmaceuticals due to lack of knowledge concerning their fate in wastes and the environment, their uptake, metabolism and excretion (pharmacokinetics) in wildlife, and their target affinity and functional effects (pharmacodynamics) in non-target species (Boxall et al., 2012). Pharmaceuticals are present in the environment as a consequence of patient use, drug production and formulation, and improper disposal (Boxall et al., 2012). They predominantly enter the aquatic environment and are typically found in concentrations from sub-ng/l to a few µg/l (aus der Beek et al., 2016). Extremely high pharmaceutical concentrations, in the order of mg/l, however, have been detected in some industrial effluents and recipient streams, for example in India, China, USA, Korea and Israel. Drugs are also found in the terrestrial environment through the application of sewage sludge to land, leaching from landfills, or irrigation of land with treated or untreated wastewaters (Nantaba et al., 2019). However, knowledge on the effects of drugs, in particular, their effects on terrestrial organisms is sparse. The contraceptive, ethinyl-estradiol (EE2), together with a range of other natural and synthetic estrogens, has been shown to cause feminisation in male fish in rivers (Jobling et al., 2006, Kidd et al., 2007, Lange et al., 2008, Lange et al., 2012). Carbamazepine is a widely used antiepileptic drug that has a potential impact on the environment due to its physico-chemical properties, which are rarely eliminated in conventional water treatment (Chen et al., 2019, Tian et al., 2019). Carbamazepine has been detected in all parts of the Baltic Sea (Björlenius et al., 2018). Laboratory studies have shown that even low concentrations of carbamazepine (10 µg L−1) are able to produce xeno-estrogenic effects in fish (Yan et al., 2018). Oxazepam at the concentration of 200 µg L^{-1} has been reported to affect wild fish behaviors implicating adverse effects on an ecological scale (Brodin et al., 2013).

2. ECOPHARMACOVIGILANCE OF NSAIDS: THE EXAPMLE OF DICLOFENAC

Eco-pharmacovigilance has been recognized as a new discipline focusing on the pharmacovigilance of the environment aiming to minimize the environmental risk of pharmaceutical pollutants (Wang et al. 2018, Wang et al., 2017, He et al., 2017). According to the World Health Organization, pharmacovigilance has been defined as "the science and activities relating to the detection, assessment understanding and prevention of adverse effects or any other possible drug related problems" (Wise et al., 2009). Thus, eco-pharmacovigilance could be defined as the science and activities associated with the detection, evaluation, understanding and prevention of adverse effects of pharmaceuticals in the environment (Velo and Moretti 2010). Eco-pharmacovigilance has many similarities with pharmacovigilance, but there are also crucial differences. The most important difference concerns signal detection in the environment as well as the difficulty in identifying cause and effect (Holm et al., 2013).

Non-steroidal anti-inflammatory drug diclofenac is one of the most commonly prescribed medicines worldwide. Thus, there is growing concern on the potential environmental risks posed by diclofenac. Chronic exposure to diclofenac may lead to severe effects for living organisms (Peltzer et al., 2019). It has been estimated that about 30-70% of diclofenac is removed through the conventional treatment system with wastewater treatment plant being the major primary sink. Thus, there is an amount of untreated diclofenac that will pass to surface water. Diclofenac can interact with other inorganic contaminants in the environment particularly in wastewater treatment plant, such as metals, organic contaminants and even with diclofenac metabolites. This process may lead to the creation of another possible emerging contaminant (Lonnappan et al., 2016).

A variety of technologies, including physical, biological, chemical as well as hybrid processes have been extensively investigated for the removal of pharmaceuticals including diclofenac from wastewater (Wang and Wang 2016, Ahmed et al., 2017). Chemical oxidation processes such as ozonation/H2O2, UV photolysis/H2O2 and photo-Fenton processes can successfully remove diclofenac (Im et al., 2013, Poul et al. 2019). Alternative elimination routes of diclofenac have been suggested such as the use of fungi such as ascomycete fungus Penicillium oxalicum as the elimination source (Olicón-Hernández Dr et al., 2019). In addition, microalgae biotechnology is a promising tool for many applications, including the elimination of nutrients and other contaminants from wastewater (Villar-Navarro et al., 2019). Thus, the use of microalgae has also been reported as an effective route for the removal of diclofenac from water (Escapa et al., 2018, Ben Ouada et al., 2019, Zhang et al., 2019, Villar-Navarro et al., 2019).

Although the environmental risk of diclofenac for freshwater has well been recognized, the environmental risk for terrestrial habitat has received less attention. The effect of diclofenac for terrestrial organisms is due to liquid or solid waste contaminated with drugs that are deposited on the land. Exposure pathways for higher vertebrates may be directly through ingestion of and contact with contaminated water, through consumption of contaminated forage, secondary exposure through predation of contaminated invertebrates and lower vertebrates, and direct exposure through coprophagy. Indeed, diclofenac can be regarded as the most representative example of adverse effect of pharmaceuticals to terrestrial organisms. Diclofenac has been shown to cause dramatic population declines (>99%) in Gyps vulture species in India and Pakistan, resulting in localised extinctions (Oaks et al., 2004, Swan et al., 2006, Taggart et al., 2007, Shore et la. 2014, Cuthbert et al., 2014, Hassan et al., 2018). Vultures are nature's most successful scavengers, and they provide an array of ecological, economic, and cultural services (Ogada et al., 2012). The decline of vultures has huge socioeconomic impact for India. Without the vultures, animal carcasses pose a threat to human health. Animal carcasses provide a potential breeding ground for numerous infectious diseases, including anthrax, and encourage the proliferation of pest species, such as rats. Population decline of vultures was due to the veterinary application of diclofenac in South-East Asia in order to treat inflammation and fever in domestic livestock. Vultures ingested diclofenac when feeding on the carcasses of livestock that had been treated with high doses shortly before their deaths. Diclofenac causes acute renal failure and death to the vultures (Green et al., 2007). In addition, diclofenac has been recognized as a threat for Spanish vultures (Margalida et al., 2014) as well as for African vultures (Naidoo et al., 2009).

Diclofenac has also been recognized as a threat for plants (Hájková et al., 2019, Kummerová et al., 2016). Diclofenac has been included in the watch list of substances in EU that requires its environmental monitoring in the member states. Diclofenac is also known to harmfully affect several environmental species already at concentrations of ≤ 1 µg/l (Vieno N, Sillanpää 2014). Although, this chapter is focused on diclofenac, the environmental risk and the necessity of eco-pharmacovigilance has been widely recognized for all the NSAIDs (He et al., 2017, Wang et al., 2017).

Apart from diclofenac, the other most frequently studied NSAIDs in terms of environmental risk, are ibuprofen, naproxen and ketoprofen (Marsik et al., 2017, Shanmugam et al., 2014). NSAIDs have been reported as one of the most dominant and frequently detected groups in environmental matrices including wastewater, surface water, suspended solids, sediments, groundwater, even drinking water. In addition, there is definitive evidence for the adverse impacts of the non-steroidal anti-inflammatory agents on scavenging birds and aquatic species (He et al., 2007, Wang et al., 2018). Ketoprofen has also been recognized as a threat for terrestrial and aquatic species (Wang et al., 2018).

3. PREDICTION OF ENVIRONMENTAL RISK

Risk is a concept common across many disciplines and depends both on exposure (e.g., frequency, timing and level of contact with a stressor) and effects (e.g., the nature and magnitude of the response to the stressor). Since the concentrations of pharmaceuticals in the environment are rather low, many researchers have doubted the ecological risk posed by pharmaceuticals. However, the truth is, that there is a luck of environmental data for a number of drugs. In addition, there are drugs with high biological potency, suggesting that even low concentrations of these drugs could be expected to have effects on non- target organisms. Predicting the exposure of non -target organisms to pharmaceuticals is quite complex. Following uptake, pharmaceuticals are metabolized to Phase I metabolites that might be more reactive that the parent drug. Currently, environmental assessments are obligatory before the approval of new drugs. Environmental assessments are conducted in parallel with phase III clinical trials. Model organisms have been used for the study of environmental risk. In addition, given that growth and developmental changes in plants induced by pharmaceuticals reflect changes in processes at the cellular and subcellular levels, cell suspension cultures have been suggested as a model for studying phytotoxicity (Svobodníková et al., 2019). In a relevant study, toxicity of diclofenac was investigated in a Nicotiana Tabacum 'Bright Yellow 2' suspension cell. The endpoints were growth and viability parameters (Svobodníková et al., 2019). Furthermore, in silico tools have been applied for the investigation of ecological risk. These include the use of models, such as quantitative structure-activity relationships (QSARs). These models can be thought as a spectrum crossing from global to local. Global models are formed from data derived from hundreds of compounds spanning broad structural classes and often mechanisms and modes of action. Although these in silico tools seem to be cost effective, they have limitations including predictions based on simple physico-chemical properties, as well as tools for grouping compounds into categories to allow for read-across. Categories can be formed using profilers for relevant interactions such as DNA or oestrogen receptor binding (Cromin et al., 2011).

4. ENVIRONMENTAL TOXICITY OF DICLOFENAC IN PLANTS

Diclofenac is one of the most commonly detected pharmaceuticals in fresh water systems. Environmental toxicity of diclofenac in plants has implications for human health. Potential human exposure to diclofenac and diclofenac metabolites through dietary intake should be taken into account (Wu et al., 2015). Diclofenac as wells as other medications and personal care products may contaminate food produce via plant uptake, thus constituting a route for human exposure (Wu et al., 2015). For example, crops may take up pharmaceuticals and personal care products through their roots (Miller et al., 2016).

The metabolism of diclofenac in plants is not well studied. Taken into account, that different plants may metabolize diclofenac differently, prediction of plant metabolites of diclofenac is not straightforward. Diclofenac is taken up by plants and undergoes rapid metabolization. According to Huber et al., already after 3h of exposure to diclofenac, diclofenac metabolites can be detected in the plant tissues. The metabolism of diclofenac in plants is similar with its metabolism in mammalian cells (Pérez and Barceló 2008). The drug is activated in a phase I reaction resulting in the hydroxylated metabolite 4'OH-diclofenac which is conjugated subsequently in phase II to a glucopyranoside, a typical plant specific metabolite (Huber et al., 2012). Diclofenac metabolism has also been studied in Arabidopsis cells. In a relevant study, Fu et al., investigated the metabolism of diclofenac in Arabidopsis cells using 14C tracing, and time-of-flight and triple quadruple mass spectrometers (Fu et al., 2017). Based on the results of this study, Phase I metabolism involved hydroxylation and successive oxidation and cyclization reactions. Phase I metabolites did not accumulate appreciably; they were instead rapidly conjugated with sulfate, glucose, and glutamic acid through Phase II metabolism. In particular, diclofenac parent was directly conjugated with glutamic acid, with acyl-glutamatyl-diclofenac accounting for >70% of the extractable metabolites after 120-h incubation. More importantly, at the end of incubation, >40% of the spiked diclofenac was in the non-extractable form, suggesting extensive sequestration into cell matter. As the authors have correctly commented, the important contribution of this study is the unravelling of unknown metabolic pathways of diclofenac including the rapid formation of non-extractable form and the dominance of diclofenac glutamate conjugate (Fu et al., 2017). In fact, the rapid conjugation of parent highlights the need to consider conjugates of emerging contaminants in higher plants, and their biological activity as well as possible implications for human health.

However, up to now, literature data is scarce in terms of ecotoxicity data especially focusing on plants as test organisms. Based on standard guidelines, ecotoxicological plant-based tests are strongly restricted due to the recommended end-points: growth and yield of plants. Relevant studies have investigated the uptake, systemic translocation, and abiotic stress responses and detoxification mechanisms induced by the exposure of plants to diclofenac (Christou et al., 2016). Lemna species are among the most important plants used for ecotoxicity testing (Alkimin et al. 2019). It has been suggested that diclofenac phytotoxicity mainly results from inhibition of photosynthesis (Majewska et al., 2018, Vannini et al., 2018).In addition, there is scarce evidence on the chronic effects of diclofenac in plants (Alkimin et al., 2019).

5. FROM ENVIRONMENTAL PHARMACOLOGY OF DICLOFENAC TO HUMAN PHARMACOLOGY OF DICLOFENAC: IMPLICATIONS FOR HUMAN HEALTH

Diclofenac is one of the most commonly prescribed drugs. Thus, there is ongoing interest on the environmental impact of human and animal use of diclofenac. Most importantly, the environmental impact of diclofenac has implications for human health. The effect of diclofenac in non-target organisms has well been documented, since diclofenac has caused dramatic population declines (>99%) in Gyps vulture species in India and Pakistan. The population decline of vultures has huge ecological consequences, as vultures are natural scavengers that eliminate animal carcasses. Unfed animal carcasses pose a threat for human health.

Another obvious link between the environmental effect of diclofenac and human health, comes from the potential effect of diclofenac into vegetables irrigated with diclofenac treated wastewater. Since global water shortage is a well-recognized problem, treated wastewater is a valuable water resource and used among others for agricultural irrigation. Thus, there is growing concern about accumulation of contaminants derived from pharmaceuticals such as diclofenac and personal care products into vegetables irrigated with treated wastewater (Wu et al., 2014). Relevant field studies have showed that the concentration levels of pharmaceuticals and personal care products identified in crops that were irrigated with treated wastewater or applied with biosolids were very low. However, potential human exposure to pharmaceuticals and personal care products through dietary intake should be taken into account. Information gaps and relevant questions for future research should be identified. (Wu et al. 2015, Prosser and Sibley 2015). Furthermore, the potential health risks from the occurrence of pharmaceuticals including diclofenac in drinking water have been investigated in different countries (Wen et al., 2014, Mohd Nasir et al., 2019, Praveena et al., 2019). The relevant studies suggested low potential health hazards for all age groups.

The example of diclofenac highlights that pharmaceuticals designed to improve human and animal health might have negative consequences from the exposure of non-target organisms. In the context of diclofenac, current knowledge on the occurrence of diclofenac in the environment should be improved (Acuña et al., 2015). Diclofenac might pose an environmental risk in freshwater as well as in treated wastewater. Potential harmful effects of diclofenac in the environment should be monitored. The discipline of environmental pharmacology should be included in the academic curriculum of medicine and the other health sciences. Clinicians should be informed on the environmental pharmacology of diclofenac. A multidisciplinary approach is needed for ensuring the environmental safety of diclofenac as well as of the other pharmaceuticals. Most importantly, involved scientists should recognize that the environmental effect of diclofenac could have direct implications for human health. Thus, the environmental pharmacology of diclofenac might link directly to the human pharmacology of diclofenac.

REFERENCES

Acuña V, Ginebreda A, Mor JR, Petrovic M, Sabater S, Sumpter J, Barceló D 2015 Balancing the health benefits and environmental risks of pharmaceuticals: *Diclofenac as an example Environ Int.* 85:327-33.

Ahmed MB, Zhou JL, Ngo HH, Guo W, Thomaidis NS, Xu J 2017 Progress in the biological and chemical treatment technologies for emerging contaminant removal from wastewater: A critical review *J Hazard Mater.* 323(Pt A):274-298.

Alkimin GD, Daniel D, Frankenbach S, Serôdio J, Soares AMVM, Barata C, Nunes B 2019 Evaluation of pharmaceutical toxic effects of non-standard endpoints on the macrophyte species Lemna minor and Lemna gibba *Sci Total Environ.* 20; 657:926-937. doi:10.1016/j.scitotenv.2018.12.002.

Alkimin GD, Daniel D, Dionísio R, Soares AMVM, Barata C, Nunes B 2019 Effects of diclofenac and salicylic acid exposure on Lemna minor: Is time a factor? *Environ Res.* 108609. doi:10.1016/j.envres.2019.108609.

Aus der Beek T, Weber FA, Bergmann A, Hickmann S, Ebert I, Hein A, Küster A 2016 Pharmaceuticals in the environment--Global occurrences and perspectives *Environ Toxicol Chem.* 35:823-35.

Ben Ouada S, Ben Ali R, Cimetiere N, Leboulanger C, Ben Ouada H, Sayadi S 2019 Biodegradation of diclofenac by two green microalgae: Picocystis sp. and Graesiella sp. *Ecotoxicol Environ Saf.* 186:109769.

Björlenius, B., Ripszám, M., Haglund, P., Lindberg, R. H., Tysklind, M., Fick, J. 2018 Pharmaceutical residues are widespread in Baltic Sea coastal and offshore waters – Screening for pharmaceuticals and modelling of environmental concentrations of carbamazepine *Sci. Total Environ.*, 633 :1496-1509.

Boxall ABA. 2009. Assessing environmental effects of human pharmaceuticals. *Toxicol. Lett.* 189, S33.

Boxall ABA, et al., 2012. Pharmaceuticals and personal care products in the environment: what are the big questions? *Environ. Health Perspect.* 120: 1221–1229.

Brodin, T., Fick, J., Jonsson, M., Klaminder, J. 2013 Dilute concentrations of a psychiatric drug alter behavior of fish from natural populations *Science* 339 :814-815.

Chen H, Gu X, Zeng Q, Mao Z 2019 Acute and Chronic Toxicity of carbamazepine on the Release of Chitobiase, Molting, and Reproduction in Daphnia similis *Int J Environ Res Public Health*. 16(2). pii: E209. doi: 10.3390/ijerph16020209.

Christou A, Antoniou C, Christodoulou C, Hapeshi E, Stavrou I, Michael C, Fatta-Kassinos D, Fotopoulos V.2016 Stress-related phenomena and detoxification mechanisms induced by common pharmaceuticals in alfalfa (Medicago sativa L.) plants *Sci Total Environ*. 557-558:652-64.

Cronin MTD, Enoch SJ, Hewitt M, Madden JC. 2011. Formation of mechanistic categories and local models to facilitate the prediction of toxicity. *ALTEX* 28: 45–49.

Cuthbert RJ, Taggart MA, Prakash V, Chakraborty SS, Deori P, Galligan T, Kulkarni M, Ranade S, Saini M, Sharma AK, Shringarpure R, Green RE.2014 Avian scavengers and the threat from veterinary pharmaceuticals Philos *Trans R Soc Lond B Biol Sci*. 369(1656).

Escapa C, Torres T, Neuparth T, Coimbra RN, García AI, Santos MM, Otero M. 2018 Zebrafish embryo bioassays for a comprehensive evaluation of microalgae efficiency in the removal of diclofenac from water. *Sci Total Environ*. 640-641:1024-1033.

Fu Q, Ye Q, Zhang J, Richards J, Borchardt D, Gan J 2017 Diclofenac in Arabidopsis cells: Rapid formation of conjugate *Environ Pollut*. 222:383-392.

Green RE, Taggart MA, Senacha KR, Raghavan B, Pain DJ, Jhala Y, Cuthbert R 2007 Oriental White-backed vulture population in India estimated from a survey of diclofenac residues in carcasses of ungulates. *PLoS ONE*. 2):e686. doi: 10.1371/journal.pone.0000686.

Hájková M, Kummerová M, Zezulka Š, Babula P, Váczi P 2019 Diclofenac as an environmental threat: Impact on the photosynthetic processes of Lemna minor chloroplasts. *Chemosphere*. 224:892-899.

Hassan IZ, Duncan N, Adawaren EO, Naidoo V. 2018 Could the environmental toxicity of diclofenac in vultures been predictable if preclinical testing methodology were applied? *Environ Toxicol Pharmacol.* 64:181-186.

He BS, Wang J, Liu J, Hu XM 2017 Eco-pharmacovigilance of non-steroidal anti-inflammatory drugs: Necessity and opportunities *Chemosphere.* 181:178-189.

Holm G, Snape JR, Murray-Smith R, Talbot J, Taylor D, Sörme P 2013 Implementing ecopharmacovigilance in practice: challenges and potential opportunities *Drug Saf.* 36:533-46.

Huber C, Bartha B, Schröder P. 2012 Metabolism of diclofenac in plants--hydroxylation is followed by glucose conjugation. *J Hazard Mater.* 243:250-256.

Im JK, Kim MK, Zoh KD 2013 Optimization of photolysis of diclofenac using a response surface methodology *Water Sci Technol.* 67:907-14.

Jobling S, Williams R, Johnson A, Taylor A, Gross-Sorokin M, Nolan M, Tyler CR, van Aerle R, Santos E, Brighty G 2006 Predicted exposures to steroid estrogens in U.K. rivers correlate with widespread sexual disruption in wild fish populations. *Environ Health Perspect.* 114 Suppl 1:32-9.

Kidd KA, Blanchfield PJ, Mills KH, Palace VP, Evans RE, Lazorchak JM, Flick RW 2007 Collapse of a fish population after exposure to a synthetic estrogen *Proc Natl Acad Sci U S A.* 104:8897-901.

Kummerová M, Zezulka Š, Babula P, Tříska J 2016 Possible ecological risk of two pharmaceuticals diclofenac and paracetamol demonstrated on a model plant Lemna minor *J Hazard Mater.* 302:351-361.

Lange A, Katsu Y, Ichikawa R, Paull GC, Chidgey LL, Coe TS, Iguchi T, Tyler CR 2008 Altered sexual development in roach (Rutilus rutilus) exposed to environmental concentrations of the pharmaceutical 17alpha-ethinylestradiol and associated expression dynamics of aromatases and estrogen receptors. *Toxicol Sci.* 106:113-23.

Lange A, Katsu Y, Miyagawa S, Ogino Y, Urushitani H, Kobayashi T, Hirai T, Shears JA, Nagae M, Yamamoto J, Ohnishi Y, Oka T, Tatarazako N, Ohta Y, Tyler CR, Iguchi T 2012 Comparative responsiveness to natural and synthetic estrogens of fish species commonly used in the laboratory and field monitoring *Aquat Toxicol.* 109:250-8.

Lonappan L, Brar SK, Das RK, Verma M, Surampalli RY 2016 Diclofenac and its transformation products: Environmental occurrence and toxicity - A review. *Environ Int.* 96:127-138.

Majewska M, Harshkova D, Guściora M, Aksmann A 2018 Phytotoxic activity of diclofenac: Evaluation using a model green alga Chlamydomonas reinhardtii with atrazine as a reference substance *Chemosphere.* 209:989-997.

Margalida A, Sánchez-Zapata JA, Blanco G, Hiraldo F, Donázar JA 2014 Diclofenac approval as a threat to Spanish vultures *Conserv Biol.* 28:631-2.

Marsik P, Rezek J, Židková M, Kramulová B, Tauchen J, Vaněk T. 2017 *Non-steroidal anti-inflammatory drugs in the watercourses of Elbe basin in Czech Republic Chemosphere.* 171:97-105.

Miller EL, Nason SL, Karthikeyan KG, Pedersen JA 2016 Root Uptake of Pharmaceuticals and Personal Care Product Ingredients *Environ Sci Technol.* 50:525-41.

Mohd Nasir FA, Praveena SM, Aris AZ 2019 Public awareness level and occurrence of pharmaceutical residues in drinking water with potential health risk: A study from Kajang (Malaysia). *Ecotoxicol Environ Saf.* 185:109681.

Naidoo V, Wolter K, Cuthbert R, Duncan N. 2009 Veterinary diclofenac threatens Africa's endangered vulture species *Regul Toxicol Pharmacol.* 53:205-8.

Nantaba F, Wasswa J, Kylin H, Palm WU, Bouwman H, Kümmerer K.2019 *Occurrence, distribution, and ecotoxicological risk assessment of selected pharmaceutical compounds in water from Lake Victoria*, Uganda Chemosphere. 239:124642.

Oaks JL, Gilbert M, Virani MZ, Watson RT, Meteyer CU, Rideout BA, Shivaprasad HL, Ahmed S, Chaudhry MJ, Arshad M, Mahmood S, Ali A, Khan AA. 2004 Diclofenac residues as the cause of vulture population decline in Pakistan *Nature* 427:630-3.

Ogada DL, Keesing F, Virani MZ.2012 Dropping dead: causes and consequences of vulture population declines worldwide *Ann N Y Acad Sci.* 1249:57-71.

Olicón-Hernández DR, Camacho-Morales RL, Pozo C, González-López J, Aranda E 2019 Evaluation of diclofenac biodegradation by the ascomycete fungus Penicillium oxalicum at flask and bench bioreactor scales *Sci Total Environ.*662:607-614.

Pohl J, Ahrens L, Carlsson G, Golovko O, Norrgren L, Weiss J, Örn S 2019 *Embryotoxicity of ozonated diclofenac, carbamazepine, and oxazepam in zebrafish (Danio rerio)* 225:191-199.

Peltzer PM, Lajmanovich RC, Martinuzzi C, Attademo AM, Curi LM, Sandoval MT Biotoxicity of diclofenac on two larval amphibians: Assessment of development, growth, cardiac function and rhythm, behavior and antioxidant system *Sci Total Environ.* 683:624-637.

Pérez S, Barceló D 2008 First evidence for occurrence of hydroxylated human metabolites of diclofenac and aceclofenac in wastewater using QqLIT-MS and QqTOF-MS. *Anal Chem.* 80:8135-45.

Pino MR, Muñiz S, Val J, Navarro E 2016 Phytotoxicity of 15 common pharmaceuticals on the germination of Lactuca sativa and photosynthesis of Chlamydomonas reinhardtii *Environ Sci Pollut Res Int.* 23:22530-22541.

Praveena SM, Mohd Rashid MZ, Mohd Nasir FA, Sze Yee W, Aris AZ. 2019 Occurrence and potential human health risk of pharmaceutical residues in drinking water from Putrajaya (Malaysia) *Ecotoxicol Environ* 180:549-556.

Prosser RS, Sibley PK. 2015 Human health risk assessment of pharmaceuticals and personal care products in plant tissue due to biosolids and manure amendments, and wastewater irrigation *Environ Int.* 75:223-33.

Santos LH, Araujo AN, Fachini A, Pena A, Delerue-Matos C, Montenegro MC. 2010. Ecotoxicological aspects related to the presence of pharmaceuticals in the aquatic environment. *J. Hazard. Mater.* 175: 45–95.

Shanmugam G, Sampath S, Selvaraj KK, Larsson DG, Ramaswamy BR 2014 Non-steroidal anti-inflammatory drugs in Indian rivers. *Environ Sci Pollut Res Int.* 21:921-31.

Shore RF, Taggart MA, Smits J, Mateo R, Richards NL, Fryday S 2014 Detection and drivers of exposure and effects of pharmaceuticals in higher vertebrates Philos *Trans R Soc Lond B Biol Sci.* 369(1656).

Svobodníková L, Kummerová M, Zezulka Š, Babula P 2019 Possible use of a Nicotiana tabacum 'Bright Yellow 2' cell suspension as a model to assess phytotoxicity of pharmaceuticals (diclofenac) *Ecotoxicol Environ Saf.* 182:109369.

Swan G, Naidoo V, Cuthbert R, Green RE, Pain DJ, Swarup D, Prakash V, Taggart M, Bekker L, Das D, Diekmann J, Diekmann M, Killian E, Meharg A, Patra RC, Saini M, Wolter K 2006 Removing the threat of diclofenac to critically endangered Asian vultures *PLoS Biol.* 2006 4:e66.

Taggart MA, Senacha KR, Green RE, Jhala YV, Raghavan B, Rahmani AR, Cuthbert R, Pain DJ, Meharg AA. 2007 Diclofenac residues in carcasses of domestic ungulates available to vultures in India *Environ Int.* 33:759-65.

Tian Y, Xia X, Wang J, Zhu L, Wang J, Zhang F, Ahmad Z. 2009 Chronic Toxicological Effects of Carbamazepine on Daphnia magna Straus: *Effects on Reproduction Traits, Body Length, and Intrinsic Growth Bull Environ Contam Toxicol.* doi: 10.1007/s00128-019-02715-w.

Velo G, Moretti U 2010 Ecopharmacovigilance for better health. Drug Saf. 33:963–968.

Vannini A, Paoli L, Vichi M, Bačkor M, Bačkorová M, Loppi S 2018 Toxicity of Diclofenac in the Fern Azolla filiculoides and the Lichen Xanthoria parietina *Bull Environ Contam Toxicol.* 100:430-437.

Vieno N, Sillanpää M 2014 Fate of diclofenac in municipal wastewater treatment plant - a review *Environ Int.* 69:28-39.

Villar-Navarro E, Baena-Nogueras RM, Paniw M, Perales JA, Lara-Martín PA. 2018 Removal of pharmaceuticals in urban wastewater: High rate algae pond (HRAP) based technologies as an alternative to activated sludge based processes *Water Res.* 139:19-29.

Wang J, Zhang M, Li S, He B 2018 Adapting and applying common methods used in pharmacovigilance to the environment: A possible starting point for the implementation of eco-pharmacovigilance. *Environ Toxicol Pharmacol*. 61:67-70.

Wang J, Zhao SQ, Zhang MY, He BS 2018 Targeted eco-pharmacovigilance for ketoprofen in the environment: Need, strategy and challenge *Chemosphere*. 194:450-462.

Wang J, He B, Yan D, Hu X 2017 Implementing ecopharmacovigilance (EPV) from a pharmacy perspective: A focus on non-steroidal anti-inflammatory drugs. *Sci Total Environ*. 603-604:772-784.

Wang J, Wang S 2016 Removal of pharmaceuticals and personal care products (PPCPs) from wastewater: *A review J Environ Manage*. 182:620-640.

Wen ZH, Chen L, Meng XZ, Duan YP, Zhang ZS, Zeng EY.2014 Occurrence and human health risk of wastewater-derived pharmaceuticals in a drinking water source for Shanghai, *East China Sci Total Environ*. 490:987-93.

Wise L, Parkinson J, Raine J, Breckenridge A. 2009 New approaches to drug safety: a pharmacovigilance tool kit. *Nat Rev Drug Discov*. 8:779–782.

Wu X, Conkle JL, Ernst F, Gan J 2014 Treated wastewater irrigation: uptake of pharmaceutical and personal care products by common vegetables under field conditions *Environ Sci Technol*. 48:11286-93.

Wu X, Dodgen LK, Conkle JL, Gan J 2015 Plant uptake of pharmaceutical and personal care products from recycled water and biosolids: *a review Sci Total Environ*. 536:655-666.

Wu X, Fu Q, Gan J 2016 Metabolism of pharmaceutical and personal care products by carrot cell cultures *Environ Pollut*. 211:141-7.

Yan, S., Wang, M., Zha, J., Zhu, L., Li, W., Luo, Q., Sun, J., Wang, Z. 2018 Environmentally Relevant Concentrations of Carbamazepine Caused Endocrine-Disrupting Effects on Nontarget Organisms, Chinese Rare Minnows (Gobiocypris rarus) *Environ. Sci. Technol*.52: 886-894.

Zhang Y, Guo J, Yao T, Zhang Y, Zhou X, Chu H 2019 The influence of four pharmaceuticals on Chlorellapyrenoidosa culture *Sci Rep*. 9:1624. doi: 10.1038/s41598-018-36609-4.

In: Environmental Pharmacology of Diclofenac ISBN: 978-1-53617-466-3
Editor: Eugenia Yiannakopoulou © 2020 Nova Science Publishers, Inc.

Chapter 6

THE ROLE OF OXIDATIVE STRESS IN THE ENVIRONMENTAL TOXICOLOGY OF DICLOFENAC

Eugenia Yiannakopoulou[*]
Department of Biomedical Sciences, Faculty of Health and Caring Sciences, University of West Attica, Athens, Greece

ABSTRACT

Diclofenac is a non steroidal anti-inflammatory agent, one of the most commonly prescribed NSAIDs worldwide. The adverse events of diclofenac in human beings are well known. In addition, diclofenac has been recognized as an environmental threat, as this pharmaceutical is often detected in waste wasters, effluents and surface waters. The mechanisms of environmental toxicity of diclofenac are not fully delineated. More importantly, the investigation of these mechanisms is methodologically demanding, as environmental toxicity of diclofenac concerns quite different organisms of the ecosystem. There are

---

[*] Corresponding Author's Email: nyiannak@teiath.gr; nyiannak@uniwa.gr.

differences in the physiology and the metabolic pathways among the different organisms. Thus, different mechanisms may be implicated in the toxicity of diclofenac in the different non target organisms. Identification of these mechanisms is crucial for the prevention as well as for the proper management of the environmental risk attributed to diclofenac. The investigational process of these mechanisms could be guided by the mechanisms of action of diclofenac in humans. It is well established, that chemicals behave as stressors and elicit stress response in different organisms. Stress response is an ubiquitous response that affects the homeostasis of all the organisms. Drugs are well recognized stressors, able to elicit the stress response. Oxidative stress has been implicated as an aetiologic factor in the pathogenesis of the toxic effects of diclofenac in humans. Therefore, it could be suggested that environmental toxicity of diclofenac to non target organisms is due to the induction of oxidative stress. Literature data suggest that oxidative stress is also implicated in the environmental toxicology of diclofenac. Modulation of oxidative stress by diclofenac has been investigated in plants as well as in aquatic organisms including Daphnia magna, zebrafish, Mediterranean mussels, and galaxiid fish. Available data suggest that diclofenac modulates oxidative stress in the different non target organisms. However, the direction of the effect is not always the same. Diclofenac behaves either as a pro-oxidant or as an antioxidant depending on the model organism and on the experimental conditions. Thus, based on existing evidence, it cannot be concluded if the environmental toxicity of diclofenac is due to the induction of oxidative stress. Given that diclofenac is a multi-target agent, it cannot be excluded that different mechanisms are implicated in the toxicity of diclofenac in the different organisms. This chapter reviews the role of oxidative stress in the environmental toxicology of diclofenac, focusing mostly on plants and on aquatic organisms. Methodological issues in the investigation of the role of oxidative stress in the environmental pharmacology of diclofenac are discussed.

Keywords: diclofenac, environmental pharmacology, oxidative stress, antioxidant enzymes

1. INTRODUCTION

Diclofenac is a non steroidal anti-inflammatory agent, one of the most commonly prescribed NSAIDs worldwide. The adverse events of diclofenac in human beings are well known. In addition, diclofenac has been recognized as an environmental threat, as this pharmaceutical is often detected in waste waters, effluents and surface waters (Pérez and Barceló 2008, Vieno and Sillanpää 2014, Acuña et al. 2015). Diclofenac has been shown to have harmful effect for several environmental species already at concentrations lower than ≤1 µg/l. Thus, there is ongoing interest on environmental pharmacology of diclofenac. Especially, there is concern on the effect of diclofenac in the aquatic environment (Pérez et al. 2008, Praskova et al. 2011, Hone et al. 2019, Bonnefille et al. 2018, Fontes et al. 2018). Importantly, diclofenac has been included in the First Watch List of the European Union Water Framework Directive in order to gather monitoring data in surface waters. At typically encountered environmental concentrations, diclofenac does not exhibit toxic effects against living organisms. However, chronic exposure to diclofenac may have severe effects.

Pollutants are commonly removed by the wastewater treatment plants, based on the activated sludge technique. However, not all compounds are removed by this technique. Furthermore, biological processes in wastewater treatment plants can convert pharmaceuticals to other thransformation products that can be more toxic than the parent compounds. It is estimated, that approximately 30-70% of diclofenac is removed through the conventional treatment system in wastewater treatment plant. According to other reports only 20%-40% of diclofenac is removed by wastewater treatment plants (Bouju et al. 2016, Vieno and Sillanpää 2014, Salgado et al. 2013, Acuña et al. 2015). In humans, diclofenac is metabolized into hydroxyl metabolites with 4'-hydroxy diclofenac (4'-OH-DCF) being the main metabolite of the phase I metabolism of diclofenac. These metabolites are excreted from the body into the aqueous environment. The untreated diclofenac passes to surface water, where it is free to interact with other inorganic contaminants in the environment particularly in wastewater treatment plant, such as metals, organic contaminants and even with metabolites of diclofenac (Lonnapan et al. 2018). Furthermore, the above interactions can lead to the production of another environmental pollutant. The same problem is encountered with another technique of diclofenac removal, the photochemical process i.e., photolysis. The combination of biological process with advanced oxidation processes has been suggested to improve the removal of diclofenac. Advanced oxidation processes include photo-Fenton, sonolysis, electrochemical oxidation, radiation and ozonation (Kanakaraju et al. 2018). These processes utilize the high reactivity of hydroxyl radicals to progressively oxidize organic compounds to innocuous products (Kanakaraju et al. 2018, Miklos et al. 2018, Dewil et al. 2017).

The mechanisms of environmental toxicity of diclofenac are not fully delineated. Identification of these mechanisms is crucial for the prevention as well as for the proper management of the environmental risk attributed to diclofenac. The investigational process of these mechanisms could be guided by the mechanisms of action of diclofenac in laboratory experimental models as well as in humans. It is well established, that chemicals behave as stressors and elicit stress response in different organisms. Stress response is an ubiquitous response that affects the homeostasis of all the organisms. Drugs are well recognized stressors, able to elicit the stress response (Yiannakopoulou et al. 2006, Yiannakopoulou 2007, Yiannakopoulou et al. 2007, Yiannakopoulou et al. 2009). Diclofenac, being a precursor of acetic acid, has been evidenced to elicit stress response in the eukaryotic organism Saccharomyces cerevisiae (Yiannakopoulou 2005, Yiannakopoulou et al. 2005). Cellular oxidative stress, results from an imbalance between pro-oxidant and anti-oxidant mechanisms due to either increased production of free oxygen radicals and/or deficiency of antioxidant mechanisms. Oxidative stress has been implicated as an aetiologic factor in the pathogenesis of the toxic effects of diclofenac in humans (Osičková et al. 2014, Galati et al. 2002). Therefore, it could be suggested that environmental toxicity of diclofenac to non target organisms is due to the induction of oxidative stress. Indeed, literature data derived from experimental studies in different organisms, suggest that oxidative stress is also implicated in the environmental toxicology of diclofenac. This chapter focuses on the role of oxidative stress in the environmental toxicology of diclofenac.

2. DICLOFENAC AND OXIDATIVE STRESS IN PLANTS

The effect of diclofenac as an environmental pollutant has been investigated in several non target organisms, including plants and fish (Matamoros et al. 2012, Majewska et al. 2018, Vanini et al. 2018). In environmental research, there are model organisms that are used for the estimation of the environmental risk of several pharmaceuticals. Lemna minor is a plant, often used as a model organism for the assessment of environmental risk of diclofenac (Alkimin et al. 2019, Kummerová et al. 2016, Matamoros et al. 2012, Cleuvers 2003). In a very recent publication, the authors, using Lemna minor as the experimental model, investigated the effect of diclofenac on photosynthesis that is an essential anabolic process (Hájková et al. 2019). The study investigated the effect of different concentrations of diclofenac on photosynthetic processes in chloroplasts isolated from Lemna minor. Oxidative stress was induced even at a concentration of 1 μM diclofenac. Importantly, diclofenac at a concentration of 10 μM increased the levels of reactive oxygen and nitrogen species while lipid peroxidation increased at a concentration of 1 μM diclofenac (Hájková et al. 2019). Regarding the functional endpoints of the study, photosynthetic processes were affected only with the highest concentrations of diclofenac (Hájková et al. 2019). In another study, in the same experimental model, 10 day exposure at different concentrations of diclofenac including 0.1, 10, and 100 μg/L was able to induce subtle changes in duckweed plant number, biomass production, and leaf area size (Kummerová et al. 2016).

Poplar plants play important role in the removal of pharmaceuticals from contaminated water. In a relevant study, Pierratini et al. investigated diclofenac uptake as well as its effect on stress enzymes activity in Populus alba Villafranca clone. Diclofenac and its metabolites were identified in the roots of the plant, already after the first day of treatment, indicating diclofenac uptake and metabolism inside the plant. Furthermore, glutathione-S-transferases increased in roots after long-term exposure to diclofenac and an increased activity of ascorbate peroxidase and glutathione reductase was detected after short and medium-term exposure to diclofenac (Pierrattini et al. 2018).

3. DICLOFENAC AND OXIDATIVE STRESS IN AQUATIC ORGANISMS

Modulation of oxidative stress by diclofenac has been investigated in different aquatic organisms, including Daphnia magna, zebrafish, Mediterranean mussels, galaxiid fish (Gómez-Oliván et al. 2014, Oliveira et al. 2015, McRae et al. 2018, McRae et al. 2019). Environmentally relevant concentrations of diclofenac have been investigated under conditions of acute or chronic exposure. Different parameters of oxidative stress have been measured including lipid peroxidation and antioxidant enzymes.

The aquatic organism, zebrafish is an aquatic model organism for the investigation of environmental toxicity of diclofenac (Hallare et al. 2004, van den Brandhof and Montforts 2010, Praskova et al. 2014, Diniz et al. 2015, Ruy et al. 2018, Praskova et al. 2019). Feito et al. reported that a very short exposure (90 min) of zebrafish embryos to 0.03 µg L−1 of diclofenac resulted in reduction of lipid peroxidation (Feito et al. 2012). Praskova et al. investigated the effect of diclofenac on oxidative stress parameters in the Zebrafish. They showed that there was no effect of diclofenac on antioxidant enzymes glutathione reductase and glutathione-S-transferase in tested fish. In addition, exposure to diclofenac resulted in reduction of lipid peroxidation in the fish (Praskova et al. 2014). On the contrary, Diniz et al. investigated the effect of diclofenac exposure and their UV photolysis by-products over seven days in adult zebrafish. Diclofenac exposure resulted in oxidative stress response, as evidenced by the increased levels of glutathione-S-transferase and catalase and the increased MDA levels corresponding to increased levels of lipid peroxidation (Diniz et al. 2015). In another study, Freitas et al. investigated the effect of exposure on diclofenac at a concentration of 1.0 µg/L on

Mytilus galloprovincialis mussels either at control temperature (17 °C) or at a raised (21 °C) temperatures for 28 days (Freitas et al. 2019). Mussels responded to both stressors, i.e., the increase in temperature and drug exposure by recruiting their antioxidant defenses. Antioxidant defences were measured by the ratio of reduced to oxidized glutathione (GSH/GSSG),. Oxidative stress damage was prevented, with the exception of diclofenac exposure at the high temperature of 21 °C. The above results indicated that diclofenac as an oxidative stressor compromised the antioxidant defences of mussels (Freitas et al. 2019). In another study focusing on the aquatic organisms, the effect of diclofenac exposure was investigated in the Mediterranean mussel Mytilus galloprovincialis and the Manila clam Ruditapes philippinarum (Munari et al. 2018). The aquatic organisms were exposed to both reduced pH and environmentally relevant concentrations of diclofenac of 0.00, 0.05 and 0.50 μg/L. Diclofenac affected the oxidative stress parameters including the antioxidant enzymes superoxide dismutase and catalase and lipid peroxidation, suggesting modulation of oxidative stress response by diclofenac (Muanri et al. 2018). In another study, Fontes et al. showed that diclofenac exposure resulted in oxidative stress and changes in antioxidant defences in the maritime organism mussel Perna Perna (Fontes et al. 2018). In that study the effects of diclofenac were also investigated in biological endpoints. Thus, exposure of the mussels to diclofenac resulted in adverse effects on fertilization rate and embryo-larval development (Fontes et al. 2018).

McRae et al. have reported that acute exposure to diclofenac elicits oxidative stress response in the galaxiid fish galaxias maculatus. The fish was exposed to two environmentally relevant concentrations of diclofenac, 0.17 μg L-1 and 763 μg L-1. Following exposure of four days, bioconcentration of diclofenac was measured in the fish and it was found to approach environmentally relevant concentrations. Oxidative stress response was measured in different organs of the fish. Diclofenac modulated oxidative stress response but not in the same direction in different organs. Thus, lipid peroxidation in the liver was significantly elevated at both concentrations but lipid peroxidation in the kidney and gill decreased after diclofenac exposure. Catalase activity was also increased in the liver of the fish, but the activity of catalase was decreased in the gill (McRae et al. 2018).

Modulation of redox homeostasis by diclofenac has also been reported in Daphnia Magna, as evidenced by the inhibition of the activity of selenium dependent glutathione peroxidases as well as the inhibition of total glutathione peroxidases (Oliveira et al. 2015). In another study, Lubiana et al. investigated the effect of diclofenac on the antioxidant system in the gills of three-spined sticklebacks (Gasterosteus aculeatus). Three-spined Sticklebacks were exposed to environmentally relevant concentrations of diclofenac, to hypoxia as well as to the combination of both stressors. Diclofenac led to suppressed catalase activity but increased gluthathione peroxidase activity. In addition, it has been reported that diclofenac at environmentally relevant concentrations affects kidney histology in three-spined sticklebacks (Näslund et al. 2017). Furthermore, exposure to diclofenac affects circadian rhythm in the same fish (Prokkola et al. 2015).

The effect of diclofenac has also been investigated in non target organisms of the common carp family (Lu et al. 2018). Diclofenac has been reported to alter oxidative stress status in the common carp as evidenced by the alterations induced in hydroperoxide content, lipid peroxidation, protein carbonyl content as well as in the activity of the antioxidant enzymes superoxide dismutase, catalase and glutathione peroxidase (Morachis-Valdez et al. 2015, Saucedo-Vence et al. 2015). In addition, Stepanova et al. reported that subchronic exposure to diclofenac (30 day toxicity), increased activity of glutathione S-transferase, and decreased activity of glutathione reductase (Stepanova et al. 2013). In the same model organism, Islas Flores et al. reported that diclofenac induced oxidative stress in the brain, liver, gill and blood of common carp as evidenced by the increased levels of lipid peroxidation and the activities of the antioxidant enzymes catalase, superoxide dismutase and glutathione peroxidase (Islas Flores et al. 2013, Islas Flores et al. 2017).

4. Discussion

The non steroidal anti-inflammatory agent diclofenac has been recognized as an environmental risk factor, able to exhibit toxicity in several non target organisms. The mechanisms by which diclofenac induced environmental toxicity are not fully delineated. Oxidative stress has been implicated as an aetiologic factor of the environmental toxicity of diclofenac in several non target organisms (Mc Rae et al. 2019). Environmentally relevant concentrations of diclofenac have been investigated in different organisms, under conditions of acute or chronic exposure. However, there are methodological issues in the measurement of oxidative stress. Different parameters of oxidative stress have been measured in different studies. However, the measurement of oxidative stress in the different studies is not standardized. Different parameters have been used for the measurement of the amount of free radicals and different biomarkers have been used for the estimation of antioxidant defences. Furthermore, there are studies that measure only the level of antioxidant defences without taking into account the level of free radicals. It should be emphasized that evaluation of cellular redox state cannot be based solely in the measurement of one or two biomarkers. A panel of biomarkers is needed for the characterization of the redox state, taken into account that there are usually methodological issues in the validity of the methods used for the measurement of these biomarkers. Measurement of biological markers of oxidative stress has not been linked with physiological processes in the majority of the studies. Linking the measurement of biological markers with physiological processes is crucial for being certain that the observed statistically significant results are also biologically meaningful.

In the majority of the studies, diclofenac has been approached as a pro-oxidant, that modulates oxidative stress in a harmful direction. However, it should be emphasized that there is also evidence of the protective effect of diclofenac as a modulator of oxidative stress.

The evidence on the protective effect of diclofenac against oxidative stress is limited. However, it is well confirmed that high concentrations of diclofenac act as a stress factor and induce cellular stress response. The toxicity of diclofenac is largely attributed to the generation of free radicals by diclofenac (Osičková et al. 2014, Galati et al. 2002). Thus, it could be expected that exposure to low concentrations of diclofenac could confer protection against lethal oxidative stress through the induction of antioxidant mechanisms. Indeed, in a relevant study, Zoubair et al. reported that diclofenac protected mice from hydroxide peroxide induced oxidative stress through the induction of antioxidant mechanisms. Oxidative stress was induced through the intraperitoneal injection of hydrogen peroxide. Diclofenac treatment increased the levels of antioxidant enzyme and restored redox homeostasis in mice (Zoubair et al. 2016).

Existing data suggest that diclofenac modulates oxidative stress in the different non target organisms. However, the direction of the effect is not always the same. Diclofenac behaves either as a pro-oxidant or as an antioxidant depending on the model organism and on the experimental conditions. Based on existing evidence, it cannot be concluded if the environmental toxicity of diclofenac is due to the induction of oxidative stress. Taking into account, that the different species are exposed to a mixture of chemicals, the investigation of the role of oxidative stress in the environmental toxicity of diclofenac becomes more complicated i.e., in the nature, non -target organisms are exposed to different chemical agents, that behave either as pro-oxidant or as anti-oxidant and thus the net effect will depend on the interaction of these agents (McRae et al. 2019).

Given that diclofenac is a multi-target agent, that modulates different cellular processes, it could be anticipated that different mechanisms could be implicated in the environmental toxicity of diclofenac. Furthermore, different mechanisms could be implicated in the environmental toxicity exhibited by diclofenac in the different non target organisms. Identification of these mechanisms is crucial for the prevention and the proper management of the environmental toxicity of diclofenac.

Conclusion

The environmental toxicity of diclofenac has been well documented. The mechanisms of this toxicity are not fully delineated. More importantly, the investigation of these mechanisms is methodologically demanding, as environmental toxicity of diclofenac concerns quite different organisms of the ecosystem. There are differences in the physiology and the metabolic pathways among the different organisms. Thus, different mechanisms may be implicated in the toxicity of diclofenac in the different non target organisms. Stress response is ubiquitous among all the species, documented even in unicellular organisms. Thus, modulation of stress response might be a common mechanism of environmental toxicity of diclofenac in all the species. Moreover, investigation of this mechanism might provide knowledge that would be meaningful for all the species. Indeed, evidence suggests, that environmentally relevant concentrations of diclofenac modulate oxidative stress in non target organisms. However, it has not been delineated if the modulation of oxidative stress is harmful or beneficial for the non target organisms. Further research is needed after standardization of the measurement of oxidative stress in the non target organisms. The possible interaction of the different pollutants should be also taken into account.

References

Acuña V, Ginebreda A, Mor JR, Petrovic M, Sabater S, Sumpter J, Barceló D 2015 Balancing the health benefits and environmental risks of pharmaceuticals: Diclofenac as an example *Environ Int.* 85:327-33.

Alkimin GD, Daniel D, Frankenbach S, Serôdio J, Soares AMVM, Barata C, Nunes B. 2019 Evaluation of pharmaceutical toxic effects of non-standard endpoints on the macrophyte species Lemna minor and Lemna gibba *Sci Total Environ.* 657:926-937.

Bonnefille B, Gomez E, Courant F, Escande A, Fenet H 2018 Diclofenac in the marine environment: A review of its occurrence and effects *Mar Pollut Bull* 131:496-506.

Bouju H, Nastold P, Beck B, Hollender J, Corvini PFX, Wintgens T 2016 Elucidation of biotransformation of diclofenac and 4′hydroxy-diclofenac during biological wastewater treatment. *J Hazard. Mater.* 301:443–452.

Cleuvers M 2003 Aquatic ecotoxicity of pharmaceuticals including the assessment of combination effects. *Toxicol Lett.* 142:185-94.

Dewil R, Mantzavinos D, Poulios I, Rodrigo MA. 2017 New perspectives for Advanced Oxidation Processes. *J. Environ. Manag.* 195:93–99.

Diniz MS, Salgado R, Pereira VJ, Carvalho G, Oehmen A, Reis MA, Noronha JP. 2015 Ecotoxicity of ketoprofen, diclofenac, atenolol and their photolysis byproducts in zebrafish (Danio rerio). *Sci Total Environ.* 505:282-9.

Feito R, Valcarcel Y, Catalá M. 2012 Biomarker assessment of toxicity with miniaturised bioassays: diclofenac as a case study. *Ecotoxicology.* 21:289–296.

Fontes MK, Gusso-Choueri PK, Maranho LA, Abessa DMS, Mazur WA, de Campos BG, Guimarães LL, de Toledo MS, Lebre D, Marques JR, Felicio AA, Cesar A, Almeida EA, Pereira CDS 2018 A tiered approach to assess effects of diclofenac on the brown mussel Perna perna: A contribution to characterize the hazard. *Water Res.* 132:361-370.

Freitas R, Coppola F, Costa S, Pretti C, Intorre L, Meucci V, Soares AMVM, Solé M. 2019 The influence of temperature on the effects induced by Triclosan and Diclofenac in mussels *Sci Total Environ.* 663:992-999.

Galati G, Tafazoli S, Sabzevari O, Chan TS, O'Brien PJ. 2002 Idiosyncratic NSAID drug induced oxidative stress. *Chem Biol Interact.* 142:25-41.

Guiloski IC, Stein Piancini LD, Dagostim AC, de Morais Calado SL, Fávaro LF, Boschen SL, Cestari MM, da Cunha C, Silva de Assis HC. 2017 Effects of environmentally relevant concentrations of the anti-inflammatory drug diclofenac in freshwater fish Rhamdia quelen. *Ecotoxicol Environ Saf.* 139:291-300.

Gómez-Oliván LM, Galar-Martínez M, García-Medina S, Valdés-Alanís A, Islas-Flores H, Neri-Cruz N 2014 Genotoxic response and oxidative stress induced by diclofenac, ibuprofen and naproxen in Daphnia magna. *Drug Chem Toxicol.* 37:391-9.

Hájková M, Kummerová M, Zezulka Š, Babula P, Váczi P 2019 Diclofenac as an environmental threat: Impact on the photosynthetic processes of Lemna minor chloroplasts *Chemosphere.* 224:892-899.

Hallare AV, Köhler H-R, Triebskorn R. 2004 Developmental toxicity and stress protein responses in zebrafish embryos after exposure to diclofenac and its solvent, DMSO. *Chemosphere* 56:659–666.

Horie Y, Yamagishi T, Yagi A, Shintaku Y, Iguchi T, Tatarazako N. 2019 The non-steroidal anti-inflammatory drug diclofenac sodium induces abnormal embryogenesis and delayed lethal effects in early life stage zebrafish (Danio rerio). *J Appl Toxicol.* 39:622-629.

Islas-Flores H, Gómez-Oliván LM, Galar-Martínez M, Colín-Cruz A, Neri-Cruz N, García-Medina S. 2013 Diclofenac-induced oxidative stress in brain, liver, gill and blood of common carp (Cyprinus carpio). *Ecotoxicol Environ Saf.* 92:32-8.

Islas-Flores H, Manuel Gómez-Oliván L, Galar-Martínez M, Michelle Sánchez-Ocampo E, SanJuan-Reyes N, Ortíz-Reynoso M, Dublán-García O. 2017 Cyto-genotoxicity and oxidative stress in common carp (Cyprinus carpio) exposed to a mixture of ibuprofen and diclofenac. *Environ Toxicol.* 32:1637-1650.

Kanakaraju D, Glass BD, Oelgemöller M. 2018 Advanced oxidation process-mediated removal of pharmaceuticals from water: A review. *J. Environ. Manag.* 219:189–207.

Kummerová M, Zezulka Š, Babula P, Tříska J. 2016 Possible ecological risk of two pharmaceuticals diclofenac and paracetamol demonstrated on a model plant Lemna minor. *J Hazard Mater.* 302:351-361.

Loise de Morais Calado S, Esterhuizen-Londt M, Cristina Silva de Assis H, Pflugmacher S. 2019 Phytoremediation: green technology for the removal of mixed contaminants of a water supply reservoir. *Int J Phytoremediation.* 21:372-379.

Lubiana P, Prokkola JM, Nikinmaa M, Burmester T, Kanerva M, Götting M. 2016 The effects of the painkiller diclofenac and hypoxia on gene transcription and antioxidant system in the gills of three-spined stickleback. *Comp Biochem Physiol C Toxicol Pharmacol.* 185-186:147-154.

Lu G, Xie Z, Zhang Z. 2018 Effects of dissolved organic matter, feeding, and water flow on the bioconcentration of diclofenac in crucian carp (Carassius auratus) *Environ Sci Pollut Res Int.* 25:7776-7784.

Lonappan L, Brar SK, Das RK, Verma M, Surampalli RY. 2016 Diclofenac and its transformation products: Environmental occurrence and toxicity - A review. *Environ Int.* 96:127-138.

Majewska M, Harshkova D, Guściora M, Aksmann A. 2018 Phytotoxic activity of diclofenac: Evaluation using a model green alga Chlamydomonas reinhardtii with atrazine as a reference substance. *Chemosphere.* 209:989-997.

Matamoros V, Nguyen LX, Arias CA, Salvadó V, Brix H 2012 Evaluation of aquatic plants for removing polar microcontaminants: a microcosm experiment. *Chemosphere.* 88:1257-64.

McRae NK, Glover CN, Burket SR, Brooks BW, Gaw S 2018 Acute exposure to an environmentally relevant concentration of diclofenac elicits oxidative stress in the culturally important galaxiid fish Galaxias maculatus *Environ Toxicol Chem.* 37:224-235.

McRae NK, Gaw S, Brooks BW, Glover CN 2019 Oxidative stress in the galaxiid fish, Galaxias maculatus, exposed to binary waterborne mixtures of the pro-oxidant cadmium and the anti-oxidant diclofenac. *Environ Pollut.* 247:638-646.

Miklos DB, Remy C, Jekel M, Linden KG, Drewes JE, Hübner U. 2018 Evaluation of advanced oxidation processes for water and wastewater treatment—A critical review. *Water Res* 139:118–131.

Munari M, Matozzo V, Gagné F, Chemello G, Riedl V, Finos L, Pastore P, Badocco D, Marin MG 2018 Does exposure to reduced pH and diclofenac induce oxidative stress in marine bivalves? A comparative study with the mussel Mytilus galloprovincialis and the clam Ruditapes philippinarum *Environ Pollut.* 240:925-937.

Morachis-Valdez G, Dublán-García O, López-Martínez LX, Galar-Martínez M, Saucedo-Vence K, Gómez-Oliván LM 2015 Chronic exposure to pollutants in Madín Reservoir (Mexico) alters oxidative stress status and flesh quality in the common carp Cyprinus carpio *Environ Sci Pollut Res Int.* 22:9159-72.

Näslund J, Fick J, Asker N, Ekman E, Larsson DGJ, Norrgren L. 2017 Diclofenac affects kidney histology in the three-spined stickleback (Gasterosteus aculeatus) at low µg/L concentrations *Aquat Toxicol.* 189:87-96.

Nkoom M, Lu G, Liu J, Dong H, Yang H 2019 Bioconcentration, behavioral, and biochemical effects of the non-steroidal anti-inflammatory drug diclofenac in Daphnia magna *Environ Sci Pollut Res Int.* 26:5704-5712.

Oliveira LL, Antunes SC, Gonçalves F, Rocha O, Nunes B 2015 Evaluation of ecotoxicological effects of drugs on Daphnia magna using different enzymatic biomarkers *Ecotoxicol Environ Saf.* 119:1 23-31.

Osičková I, Banďouchová H, Kováčová V, Král J, Novotný L, Ondráček K, Pohanka M, Sedláčková J, Škochová H, Vitula F, Pikula J 2014 Oxidative stress and liver damage in birds exposed to diclofenac and lead *Acta Vet. BRNO* 83: 299–304.

Pérez S, Barceló D. 2008 First evidence for occurrence of hydroxylated human metabolites of diclofenac and aceclofenac in wastewater using QqLIT-MS and QqTOF-MS. *Anal Chem.* 80:8135-45.

Pierattini EC, Francini A, Huber C, Sebastiani L, Schröder P 2018 Poplar and diclofenac pollution: A focus on physiology, oxidative stress and uptake in plant organs *Sci Total Environ.* 636:944-952.

Praskova E, Voslarova E, Siroka Z, Plhalova L, Macova S, Marsalek P, Pistekova V, Svobodova Z. 2019 Assessment of diclofenac LC50 reference values in juvenile and embryonic stages of the zebrafish (Danio rerio). *Pol J Vet Sci* 14 :545-9.

Praskova E, Plhalova L, Chromcova L, Stepanova S, Bedanova I, Blahova J, Hostovsky M, Skoric M, Maršálek P, Voslarova E, Svobodova Z. 2014 Effects of subchronic exposure of diclofenac on growth, histopathological changes, and oxidative stress in zebrafish (Danio rerio). *Scientific World Journal* 2014:645737. doi: 10.1155/2014/645 737.

Prokkola JM, Nikinmaa M, Lubiana P, Kanerva M, McCairns RJ, Götting M 2015 . Hypoxia and the pharmaceutical diclofenac influence the circadian responses of three-spined stickleback *Aquat Toxicol.* 158:11 6-24.

Ryu B, Kim CY, Oh H, Kim U, Kim J, Jung CR, Lee BH, Lee S, Chang SN, Lee JM, Chung HM, Park JH. 2018 Development of an alternative zebrafish model for drug-induced intestinal toxicity *J Appl Toxicol.* 38:259-273.

Salgado R., Pereira V. J., Carvalho G., Soeiro R., Gaffney V., Almeida C., Cardoso V. V., Ferreira E., Benoliel M. J., Ternes T. A., et al. Photodegradation kinetics and transformation products of ketoprofen, diclofenac and atenolol in pure water and treated wastewater. *J. Hazard. Mater.* 2013;244–245:516–527.

Saucedo-Vence, K., Dublán-García, O., López-Martínez, L. X., Morachis-Valdes, G., Galar-Martínez, M., Islas-Flores, H., Gómez-Oliván, L. M. 2015 Short and long-term exposure to diclofenac alter oxidative stress status in common carp Cyprinus carpio *Ecotoxicology.* 24:527-39.

Stepanova, S., Praskova, E., Chromcova, L., Plhalova, L., Prokes, M., Blahova, J, Svobodova, Z. 2013 The effects of diclofenac on early life stages of common carp (Cyprinus carpio). *Environ Toxicol Pharmacol.* 35:454-60.

Trombini, C., Hampel, M., Blasco, J. 2019 Assessing the effect of human pharmaceuticals (carbamazepine, diclofenac and ibuprofen) on the marine clam Ruditapes philippinarum: An integrative and multibiomarker approach *Aquat Toxicol.* 208:146-156.

Van den Brandhof, E-J., Montforts, M. 2010 Fish embryo toxicity of carbamazepine, diclofenac and metoprolol. *Ecotoxicology and Environmental Safety.* 73:1862–1866.

Vannini, A., Paoli, L., Vichi, M., Bačkor, M., Bačkorová, M., Loppi, S. 2018 Toxicity of Diclofenac in the Fern Azolla filiculoides and the Lichen Xanthoria parietina. *Bull Environ Contam Toxicol.* 100:430-437.

Vieno, N., Sillanpää, M. 2014 Fate of diclofenac in municipal wastewater treatment plant - a review. *2014 Environ Int.* 69:28-39.

Yiannakopoulou, E. 2005 *Cellular mechanisms of adaptation in oxidative stress and in heat shock in Saccharomyces cerevisiae: the effect of antioxidants* Msc Thesis for the Msc Medical Biology Medical School and Department of Biology University of Athens.

Yiannakopoulou, E. Ch., Delitheos, A., and Tiligada, E. 2005 Dose-dependent effect of non-steroidal anti-inflammatory agents on the cellular stress response. *Epitheor Klin Farmacol Farmakokinet* 23: 39–41.

Yiannakopoulou, E., 2007 Investigation of the role of salicylates in preconditioning *Final Report for Postdoctoral Research* (IKY Scholarship 15109/07.10.2005).

Yiannakopoulou, ECh., and Tiligada, E. 2007 Pharmacological preconditioning in the oxidative stress response of eukaryotic cells: In process method validation. *Epitheor Klin Farmacol Farmakokinet* 25: 30–32.

Yiannakopoulou E., Tiligada E., 2009 Preconditioning effect of salicylates against oxidative stress in yeast. *J Appl Microbiol* 106:903-908.

Yiannakopoulou ECh., Tiligada, E., 2006 Acetaminophen modulates the oxidative stress response in eucaryotic cells. *Rev Clin Pharmacol Pharmacokinet* 20: 125–127.

Zezulka, Š., Kummerová, M., Babula, P., Hájková, M., Oravec, M. 2019 Sensitivity of physiological and biochemical endpoints in early ontogenetic stages of crops under diclofenac and paracetamol treatments *Environ Sci Pollut Res Int.* 26:3965-3979.

Zoubair, B., Azzahra, L. F., Fouzia, H., Mohammed, L., Brahim, B., Noureddine B. 2016 Evaluation of Diclofenac effect on oxidative stressed mice, *Int. J. Pure App. Biosci.* 4: 1-8

In: Environmental Pharmacology of Diclofenac ISBN: 978-1-53617-466-3
Editor: Eugenia Yiannakopoulou © 2020 Nova Science Publishers, Inc.

Chapter 7

METHODOLOGICAL ISSUES IN ENVIRONMENTAL PHARMACOLOGY: THE PARADIGM OF DICLOFENAC

*Eugenia Yiannakopoulou**
Department of Biomedical Sciences, Faculty of Health Sciences,
University of West Attica, Athens, Greece

ABSTRACT

Environmental pharmacology is a developing science that investigates potential adverse effects of drugs in the environment. Currently, there is concern on the potential impact of pharmaceuticals in the environment. There are examples of drugs with well documented adverse effects in the environment. The veterinary use of the non steroidal anti-inflammatory agent diclofenac has led to a dramatically huge population decline of Gyps vultures in India and Pakistan. On the other hand, the drug 17α-ethinylestradiol has been implicated in fish feminization. Thus, the environmental risk assessment has been

---

* Corresponding Author's Email: nyiannak@teiath.gr; nyiannak@uniwa.gr.

introduced as a regulatory requirement before the approval of a new drug. However, environmental risk assessment does not always reflect real life, as it is conducted in the laboratory and concerns a limited number of species. Additionally, it is doubtful if these regulatory controls reflect the risk of the different environmental species. Potentially all species in the environment including humans could be exposed to a new drug. More importantly, adverse environmental impact can be caused by old drugs. The example of diclofenac highlights the environmental risk that could be attributed to the old drugs. Thus, actions are needed for the standardized monitoring of the environmental impact of old drugs. Identifying the potential adverse environmental impact of a drug is a laborious process that shares common points with the identification of adverse drug reactions. However, the investigation of the environmental impact of a drug is quite more demanding and a multidisciplinary approach is needed. Furthermore, diverse methodological issues have been raised, that are derived from the diversity of environmental species as well as from the potential exposure of these species to multiple drugs and chemicals. Appropriate bioassays should be applied. The effect of chronic exposure should be systematically evaluated. The combined effect of different pharmaceuticals should be taken into account. The combined effect of adverse environmental conditions in combination with exposure to pharmaceuticals should also be investigated. Undoubtedly, there is lack of experimental data to contribute knowledge on the potential effect of all pharmaceuticals to the diverse non target organisms. Furthermore, gathering and analysing these data is also demanding. Computational tools such as quantitative structure toxicity relationship could fill the gap and contribute to an integrated approach. This chapter is focused on the above mentioned methodological issues that are approached through the example of diclofenac. The chapter is structured in five sections including a section that introduces the reader to the methodological issues araised in the environmental pharmacology research, the second section concerns studies of acute toxicity, the third section is focused on methodological issues of chronic toxicity studies, the fourth section presents the difficulties arising due to the exposure of non target organisms to multiple agents and the fifth section presents implications for further research.

Keywords: diclofenac, environmental pharmacology, methodological issues, environmental pharmacology of mixtures, in silico approaches

1. INTRODUCTION

Environmental pharmacology is a developing science that investigates potential adverse effects of drugs in the environment. Currently, there is concern on the potential impact of pharmaceuticals in the environment. There are examples of drugs with well documented adverse effects in the environment. The veterinary use of the non steroidal anti-inflammatory agent diclofenac has led to a dramatically huge population decline of Gyps vultures in India and Pakistan (Green et al. 2007). On the other hand, 17α-ethinyl-estradiol .has been implicated in male fish feminization in rivers (Jobling et al. 2006, Kidd et al. 2007, Lange et al., 2008, Lange et al. 2012). Thus, the environmental risk assessment has been introduced as a regulatory requirement before the approval of a new drug. However, environmental risk assessment dose not always reflect real life, as it is conducted in the laboratory and concerns a limited number of species. Additionally, it is doubtful if these regulatory controls reflect the risk of the different environmental species. Potentially all species in the environment including humans could be exposed to a new drug. More importantly, adverse environmental impact can be caused by old drugs. The example of diclofenac highlights the environmental risk that could be attributed to the old drugs. Thus, actions are needed for the standardized monitoring of the environmental impact of old drugs. Identifying the potential adverse environmental impact of a drug is a laborious process that shares common points with the identification of adverse drug reactions. However, the investigation of the environmental impact of a drug is quite more demanding and a multidisciplinary approach is needed. Furthermore, diverse methodological issues are raised, that are derived from the diversity of environmental species as well as from the potential exposure of these species to multiple drugs and chemicals. This chapter is focused on these methodological issues that are approached through the example of diclofenac.

2. ACUTE EXPOSURE

The potential toxic effect of environmental exposure to diclofenac has been investigated in different organisms. A significant number of acute toxicity studies have examined the environmental effect of diclofenac in aquatic organisms, due to wide detection of diclofenac in surface water worldwide (Hallare et al. 2004, van den Brandhof et al. 2010, Feito et al. 2012, Ribas et al. 2017, Ghelfi et al. 2016, McRae et al. 2018). Studies of acute toxicity have also evaluated the potential toxic effect of diclofenac in plants (Alkimin et al. 2019). In these studies, the exposure lasts for a few hours up to about 96 hours. Different concentrations of diclofenac have been investigated. Studies of acute exposure could be implemented easily due to low cost and low level of resources. Although, these studies contribute knowledge on the environmental risk of diclofenac, it is doubtful if this knowledge is biologically useful, as the exposure of different species to pharmaceuticals and chemical agents lasts for years. However, the studies of acute exposure could be seen as hypothesis generating with the aim to study these hypotheses to subsequent studies of chronic exposure. The studies of acute exposure could guide the design and methodology of chronic exposure studies.

3. CHRONIC EXPOSURE

Commonly, environmental effects of pharmaceuticals are often studied and observed at non-environmentally relevant concentrations of single compounds via acute toxicity bioassays that are conducted under defined laboratory conditions (Carlsson 2006). Non target organisms are often submitted to chronic exposure to pharmaceuticals. Although there are numerous studies that investigate the environmental risk of pharmaceuticals under short term conditions, it is quite difficult to monitor the effects of the chronic exposure. More importantly, it is difficult to predict if applied research methodology represents real life. Commonly the effect of chronic exposure to pharmaceuticals is investigated in experimental non target organisms via chronic toxicity bioassays of several days (Charry et al. 2019, Liu et al. 2019, Wang et al. 2016, Dahms et al. 2016, Stringer et al. 2014). Appropriate experimental organisms should be widely distributed and ecologically important, play an important role in the transportation of pollutants across the food chain and also allow the application of whole animal assays as well as of gene expression studies (Raisuddin et al. 2007). Although, it is essential to standardise a battery of test organisms from species in different phylogenetic and critical ecosystem positions, it is unclear if the potential effect of pharmaceuticals on these experimental organisms could capture the potential effect on all the diverse organisms and especially on wildlife organisms. Furthermore, it should be taken into account that the effect of a pharmaceutical in some non-target organisms might be idiosyncratic. Thus, it has been suggested that the effect of diclofenac in vultures is idiosyncratic, as a result of the metabolism specific to species (Hassan et al. 2018).

Thus, studies focusing on the potential effect of pharmaceuticals on plants are scarce (Alkimin et al. 2019), as the recommended standard endpoints of growth and yield of plants are difficult to be implemented (Alkimin et al. 2019). Furthermore, it is doubtful if a chronic toxicity test of several days could reflect the effect of chronic exposure to pharmaceuticals over years. Chronic exposure is defined differently in the different studies, thus there are authors that investigate the effect of chronic exposure through bioassays of 21 days and others that define as sub-chronic exposure the bio-assay of 28 days duration (Guilioski et al. 2017, Praskova et al. 2014). The duration of a three month of exposure of fish to diclofenac has also been defined as chronic exposure (Lee et al. 2011).

The bioassays that investigate the environmental effect of pharmaceuticals should be also standardized and especially adopted to the mechanisms of action of the different pharmaceuticals as wells as to the physiology of different organisms. Not all bioassays are suitable for all the non target organisms. Commonly, the studies that investigate the environmental effect of pharmaceuticals include endpoints of survival, growth rate, reproduction, embryonic development. In addition, the effect in biochemical markers is also investigated. Methodologically, a number of issues have been raised. First of all, it is questionable if environmentally relevant concentrationse are the same for the different organisms. Second, chronic exposure might be differently defined in the different organisms. Third, in the majority of the studies multiple endpoints are investigated in the same study without taking into account the possibility of false statistically significant effect due to multiple comparisons.

In the case of diclofenac, it has been shown that chronic exposure to diclofenac modulates the reproductive physiology of fish by altering the expression of important key enzymes of the hypothalamus-pituitary-gonad-axis and might act as an estrogenic endocrine disrupting chemical (Gröner et al. 2015, . Gröner et al. 2017, Effosa et al. 2017). In another relevant study Mezzelani et al. investigated the molecular and cellular effects of diclofenac in mussels Mytilus galloprovincialis exposed to the realistic environmental concentration of 2.5 µg/L for up to 60 days. The results showed a significant accumulation of diclofenac and also alterations of immunological parameters, genotoxic effects, modulation of lipid metabolism and changes in cellular turn-over caused by the chronic exposure to diclofenac (Mezzelani et al. 2018). Adverse effects of chronic exposure to diclofenac on aquatic invertebrates have also been reported in other studies (Nieto et al. 2017, Liu et al. 2017). Liu et al. investigated the effects of diclofenac on survival, growth rate and reproduction of the aquatic invertebrate Daphnia magna via a 21 days chronic toxicity test. Based on the results, the reproduction parameters were adversely affected by the chronic toxicity test (Liu et al. 2017). In the same study, the authors also investigated the effects of diclofenac on the expression of the genes related to the detoxification metabolism, growth, development and reproduction of Daphnia magna, e.g., HR96, P-gp, CYP360A8, CYP314, GST, EcR and Vtg though an acute exposure test of up to 96h. Gene expression was affected by the diclofenac exposure and the effect was dose and time dependent (Liu et al). Guiloski et al. have investigated the effect of chronic exposure to diclofenac of the fish Rhamdia quelen via a bioassay of 21 days (Guilioski et al. 2017). The fish were exposed to environmental concentrations of diclofenac of 0, 0.2, 2 and 20µg/L.

Potential biochemical, genetic and reproductive effects of diclofenac were studied. In the liver, diclofenac reduced the activities of antioxidant enzymes catalase and superoxide dismutase. In addition, diclofenac increased the activities of glutathione and glutathione transferase. However, these results are difficult to be interpreted. Mechanistically, the effect of diclofenac should be the same in all the tested antioixdants. Lipid peroxidation was reduced in the groups exposed to 0.2 and 20 µg/l. However, the concentration of 2 µg/L would be expected to have also the same effect. In the testis, exposure to the concentration of 0.2 µg/L resulted in inhibition of superoixe dismutase, glutathione peroxidase and glutathione transferase activities (Guiloski et al. 2017). The question still arises why the concentrations of 2µg/L as well as the concentration of 20 µg/L did not affect anti-oxidant enzymes in the testis. The above questions underscore the necessity of strict adoption of basic principles of human pharmacology in the environmental pharmacology. Thus, a clinically significant effect should be expected to be dose-dependent and time-dependent in order to be meaningful.

Histopathological alterations in organs of non target organisms induced by chronic exposure to diclofenac have also been reported (Hoeger et al. 2005, Schwaiger et al. 2004). In a relevant study, Schweiger et al, investigated the effect of diclofenac exposure to tissues of the rainbow trout (Oncorhynchus mykiss), exposed to diclofenac concentrations ranging from 1 µg L−1 to 500 µg L−1 over a 28-day period (Schweiger et al. 2004). The highest concentrations of diclofenac were found in the liver, followed by the kidneys and the gills. The most prominent effects of diclofenac in the kidney included a severe accumulation of protein in the tubular cells, macrophage infiltration, and structural alterations i.e dilation and vesiculation of the endoplasmic reticulum in the renal tubules, necrosis of endothelial cells in the renal corpuscles. In the liver, collapse of the cellular compartmentation and glycogen depletion in hepatocytes were observed.

4. MULTIPLE AGENTS

In human pharmacology, it is well recognized that supporting a casual relationship between a drug, or a combination of drugs and an adverse reaction is not always straightforward. In environmental pharmacology, attributing adverse environmental impacts on environmental species to a single cause such as an individual drug, combination of drugs or a drug metabolite is really complicated (Rand-Weaver 2013). The different environmental species are exposed to an array of diverse chemicals as well as to other adverse environmental factors. Thus, it is difficult to identify which drug, chemical or environmental factor is responsible for an adverse environmental impact. Furthermore, it is quite common that the observed effect represented the combined effect of a mixture of pharmaceuticals or the combined effect of a pharmaceutical and an adverse condition. In the case of diclofenac, the combined effect of an adverse condition i.e., acidified water, elevated temperature with diclofenac exposure have been examined in a number of studies. (Freitas et al. 2019, McRae et al. 2019, Munari et al. 2018, Munari et al. 2016). In a recent study, Munari et al. investigated the combined effects of seawater acidification and of diclofenac exposure on haemocyte parameters of the mussel Mytilus galloprovincialis and the clam Ruditapes philippinarum. Examined hemocyte parameters included total haemocyte count, haemocyte volume and diameter, neutral Red uptake, haemocyte proliferation and lysozyme activity. The above mentioned parameters were measured after 7, 14 and 21 days of exposure to differing pH value or pH/diclofenac combinations (Munari et al. 2019). A synergistic interaction between pH and diclofenac was observed in mussels that affected mainly hemocyte size and lysozyme activity (Munari et al. 2019).

It is well recognized that environmental contaminants are commonly encountered as mixtures, and the behaviour of chemicals in a mixture may not correspond to that predicted from data on the pure compounds (Altenburger et al. 2003). It is well known, that interactions of components in a mixture can cause complex and substantial changes in the apparent properties of its constituents, resulting in synergistic or antagonistic effects

Thus, in the case of diclofenac the combined effect of environmental exposure to diclofenac and another pharmaceutical or another chemical substance has also been studied (Schmidt et al. 2011, Osickova et al. 2012, Schmidt et al. 2014, Doležalová Weissmannová et al. 2018, Ukić et al. 2019). Environmental toxicity data for mixtures of pharmaceuticals are quite scarce. Investigation of the environmental toxicity of mixtures of pharmaceuticals is really demanding as toxicity data vary with different combinations the same chemicals in a mixture and furthermore complex interactions exist among different chemicals. Thus, it is quite difficult to design animal and in vitro studies for the study of environmental toxicity of pharmaceuticals. Computational approaches are promising alternative solutions for studying the environmental toxicity of mixtures of pharmaceuticals. In silico methods like quantitative structure activity relationships (QSAR) and machine learning (ML) approaches trained on experimental data could be beneficial for the making predictions for the environmental toxicity of mixtures of pharmaceuticals (Zhou et al. 2011, Toropova et al. 2012, Tang et al. 2013, Yao et al. 2013, Wang et al. 2016). The above mentioned computational methods are able to model the relationships between toxicity and drug or chemical properties based on chemical structure and physicochemical properties. Of course, experimental data are needed as input parameters for the training of computational approaches. The results of computational methods should also be verified by in vivo experimental data.

5. IMPLICATIONS FOR FURTHER RESEARCH

Monitoring of the potential adverse environmental impact of old and novel drugs should be standardized. The potential adverse environmental effect of pharmaceuticals should be investigated in different laboratory organisms that are well validated and representative of the different ecosystems. Appropriate bioassays should be applied. The effect of chronic exposure should be systematically evaluated. The combined effect of different pharmaceuticals should be taken into account. The combined effect of adverse environmental conditions in combination with exposure to pharmaceuticals should also be investigated. The mechanisms underlying the environmental toxicity of pharmaceuticals should be thoroughly investigated. Targeted ecopharmacovigilance will contribute to the recognition of the potential risk for the environment and lead further research. Targeted eco-pharmacovigilance that focuses on individual or specific pharmaceuticals on a prioritised basis is a feasible, economical and customized approach to reduce the environmental concentrations and risks of pharmaceuticals (Wang et al. 2017, Wang et al. 2018). It should be kept in mind that monitoring should include all environmental species including terrestrial and aquatic species.

Undoubtedly, there is lack of experimental data to contribute knowledge on the potential effect of all pharmaceuticals to the diverse non target organisms. Furthermore, gathering and analysing these data is also demanding. Computational tools such as quantitative structure toxicity relationship could fill the gap and contribute to an integrated approach (Khan et al. 2018). Thus, in silico approaches should be developed and validated for mining of big data derived from untargeted methods (Kar et al. 2018, Kar and Leszczynski 2019).

REFERENCES

Alkimin, G. D., Daniel, D., Dionísio, R., Soares, A. M. V. M., Barata, C., Nunes, B., 2019 Effects of diclofenac and salicylic acid exposure on Lemna minor: Is time a factor? *Environ Res.* 177:108609.

Alkimin, G. D., Daniel, D., Frankenbach, S., Serôdio, J., Soares, A. M. V. M., Barata, C., Nunes, B. 2019 Evaluation of pharmaceutical toxic effects of non-standard endpoints on the macrophyte species Lemna minor and Lemna gibba. *Sci Total Environ.* 657:926-937.

Altenburger, R., Nendza, M., Schüürmann, G. 2003 Mixture toxicity and its modeling by quantitative structure-activity relationships. *Environ Toxicol Chem.* 22:1900-15.

Alkimin, G. D., Daniel, D., Frankenbach, S., Serôdio, J., Soares, A. M. V. M., Barata, C., Nunes, B. 2019 Evaluation of pharmaceutical toxic effects of non-standard endpoints on the macrophyte species Lemna minor and Lemna gibba. *Sci Total Environ.* 657:926-937.

Carlsson, C. 2006 Are pharmaceuticals potent environmental pollutants? *Sci. Total Environ.* 364:67–87.

Charry, M. P., Northcott, G. L., Gaw, S., Keesing, V., Costello, M. J., Tremblay, L. A. 2019 Development of acute and chronic toxicity bioassays using the pelagic copepod Gladioferens pectinatus. *Ecotoxicol Environ Saf.* 174:611-617.

Dahms, H. U., Won, E. J., Kim, H. S., Han, J., Park, H. G., Souissi, S., Raisuddin, S., Lee, J. S. 2016 Potential of the small cyclopoid copepod Paracyclopina nana as an invertebrate model for ecotoxicity testing. *Aquat Toxicol* 180:282-294.

Doležalová Weissmannová, H., Pavlovský, J., Fišerová, L., Kosárová, H. 2018 Toxicity of Diclofenac: Cadmium Binary Mixtures to Algae Desmodesmus subspicatus Using Normalization Method. *Bull Environ Contam Toxicol.* 101:205-213.

Efosa, N. J., Kleiner, W., Kloas, W., Hoffmann, F. 2017 Diclofenac can exhibit estrogenic modes of action in male Xenopus laevis, and affects the hypothalamus-pituitary-gonad axis and mating vocalizations. *Chemosphere.* 173:69-77.

Feito, R., Valcarcel, Y., Catalá, M. 2012 Biomarker assessment of toxicity with miniaturised bioassays: diclofenac as a case study. *Ecotoxicology.* 21:289–296.

Freitas, R., Coppola, F., Costa, S., Pretti, C., Intorre, L., Meucci, V., Soares, A. M. V. M., Solé, M. 2019 The influence of temperature on the effects induced by Triclosan and Diclofenac in mussels. *Sci Total Environ.* 663:992-999.

Freitas, R., Coppola, F., Costa, S., Manzini, C., Intorre, L., Meucci, V., Soares, A. M. V. M., Pretti, C., Solé, M. 2019 Does salinity modulates the response of Mytilus galloprovincialis exposed to triclosan and diclofenac? *Environ Pollut.* 251:756-765.

Ghelfi, A., Ribas, J. L., Guiloski, I. C., Bettim, F. L., Piancini, L. D., Cestari, M. M., Pereira, A. J., Sassaki, G. L., Silva de Assis, H. C. 2016 Evaluation of Biochemical, Genetic and Hematological

Biomarkers in a Commercial Catfish Rhamdia quelen Exposed to Diclofenac. *Bull Environ Contam Toxicol.* 96:49-54.

Guiloski I. C., Stein Piancini, L.D, Dagostim, A.C., de Morais Calado, S. L., Fávaro, L. F., Boschen, S. L., Cestari, M. M., da Cunha, C., Silva de Assis, H. C. 2017 Effects of environmentally relevant concentrations of the anti-inflammatory drug diclofenac in freshwater fish Rhamdia quelen. *Ecotoxicol Environ Saf.* 139:291-300.

Green, R. E., Taggart, M. A., Senacha, K. R., Raghavan, B., Pain, D. J., Jhala, Y., Cuthbert, R. 2007 Oriental White-backed vulture population in India estimated from a survey of diclofenac residues in carcasses of ungulates. *PLoS ONE.* 2):e686. doi: 10.1371/journal.pone.0000686.

Gröner F, Höhne C, Kleiner W, Kloas W 2017 Chronic diclofenac exposure affects gill integrity and pituitary gene expression and displays estrogenic activity in nile tilapia (Oreochromis niloticus). *Chemosphere* 166:473-481.

Gröner, F., Höhne, C., Kleiner, W., Kloas, W. 2017 Chronic exposure to the ß-blocker metoprolol reduces growth and alters gene expression of gonadotropins and vitellogenin in Nile tilapia (Oreochromis niloticus). *Ecotoxicol Environ Saf.* 141:271-279.

Gröner, F., Ziková, A., Kloas, W. 2015 Effects of the pharmaceuticals diclofenac and metoprolol on gene expression levels of enzymes of biotransformation, excretion pathways and estrogenicity in primary hepatocytes of Nile tilapia (Oreochromis niloticus). *Comp Biochem Physiol C Toxicol Pharmacol.* 167:51-57.

Guyon, A., Smith, K. F., Charry, M. P., Champeau, O., Tremblay, L. A. 2018 Effects of chronic exposure to benzophenone and diclofenac on DNA methylation levels and reproductive success in a marine copepod. *J Xenobiot.* 2018 8:7674.

Hallare, A. V., Köhler, H-R., Triebskorn, R. 2004 Developmental toxicity and stress protein responses in zebrafish embryos after exposure to diclofenac and its solvent, DMSO. *Chemosphere.* 56:659–666.

Hassan, I. Z., Duncan, N., Adawaren, E. O., Naidoo V 2018 Could the environmental toxicity of diclofenac in vultures been predictable if preclinical testing methodology were applied? *Environ Toxicol Pharmacol.* 64:181-186.

Hoeger, B. 1, Köllner, B., Dietrich, D. R., Hitzfeld, B. 2005 Water-borne diclofenac affects kidney and gill integrity and selected immune parameters in brown trout (Salmo trutta f. fario). *Aquat Toxicol.* 75:53-64.

Hossain, K. A., Roy, K. 2018 Chemometric modeling of aquatic toxicity of contaminants of emerging concern (CECs) in Dugesia japonica and its interspecies correlation with daphnia and fish: QSTR and QSTTR approaches. *Ecotoxicol Environ Saf.* 166:92-101.

Jobling, S., Williams, R., Johnson, A., Taylor, A., Gross-Sorokin, M., Nolan, M., Tyler, C. R., van Aerle, R., Santos, E., Brighty, G. 2006 Predicted exposures to steroid estrogens in U.K. rivers correlate with widespread sexual disruption in wild fish populations. *Environ Health Perspect.* 114 Suppl 1:32-9.

Kar, S., Leszczynski, J. 2019 Exploration of Computational Approaches to Predict the Toxicity of Chemical Mixtures Toxics. 7. pii: E15. doi: 10.3390/toxics7010015.

Kar, S., Roy, K., Leszczynski, J. 2018 Impact of Pharmaceuticals on the Environment: Risk Assessment Using QSAR Modeling Approach. *Methods Mol Biol* 1800:395-443.

Khan, K., Kar, S., Sanderson, H., Roy, K., Leszczynski, J. 2018 Ecotoxicological Modeling, Ranking and Prioritization of Pharmaceuticals Using QSTR and i-QSTTR Approaches: Application of 2D and Fragment Based Descriptors. *Mol Inform.* doi: 10.1002/minf.2018 00078.

Kidd, K. A., Blanchfield, P. J., Mills, K. H., Palace, V. P., Evans, R. E., Lazorchak, J. M., Flick, R. W. 2007 Collapse of a fish population after exposure to a synthetic estrogen. *Proc Natl Acad Sci U S A.* 104:8897-901.

Lange, A., Katsu, Y., Ichikawa, R., Paull, G. C., Chidgey, L. L., Coe, T. S., Iguchi T., Tyler C. R. 2008 Altered sexual development in roach (Rutilus rutilus) exposed to environmental concentrations of the pharmaceutical 17alpha-ethinylestradiol and associated expression dynamics of aromatases and estrogen receptors. *Toxicol Sci.* 106:113-23.

Lange, A., Katsu, Y., Miyagawa S., Ogino Y., Urushitani, H., Kobayashi, T., Hirai, T., Shears, J. A., Nagae, M., Yamamoto, J., Ohnishi, Y., Oka, T., Tatarazako, N., Ohta, Y., Tyler, C. R., Iguchi, T. 2012 Comparative responsiveness to natural and synthetic estrogens of fish species commonly used in the laboratory and field monitoring. *Aquat Toxicol.* 109:250-8.

Lee, J., Ji, K., Lim Kho, Y., Kim, P., Choi, K. 2011 Chronic exposure to diclofenac on two freshwater cladocerans and Japanese medaka. *Ecotoxicology and Environmental Safety.* 74:1216–1225.

Liu, Y., Wang, L., Pan, B., Wang, C., Bao, S., Nie, X. 2017 Toxic effects of diclofenac on life history parameters and the expression of detoxification-related genes in Daphnia magna. *Aquat Toxicol.* 183:104-113.

Liu, Y., Ding, R., Pan, B., Wang, L., Liu, S., Nie, X. 2019 Simvastatin affect the expression of detoxification-related genes and enzymes in Daphnia magna and alter its life history parameters. *Ecotoxicol Environ Saf.* 182:109389.

McRae, N. K., Glover, C. N., Burket, S. R., Brooks, B. W., Gaw, S. 2018 Acute exposure to an environmentally relevant concentration of diclofenac elicits oxidative stress in the culturally important galaxiid fish Galaxias maculatus. *Environ Toxicol Chem.* 37:224-235.

McRae, N. K., Gaw, S., Brooks, B. W., Glover, C. N. 2019 Oxidative stress in the galaxiid fish, Galaxias maculatus, exposed to binary waterborne mixtures of the pro-oxidant cadmium and the anti-oxidant diclofenac *Environ Pollut.* 247:638-646.

Mezzelani, M., Gorbi, S., Fattorini, D., d'Errico, G., Consolandi, G., Milan, M., Bargelloni, L., Regoli, F. 2018 Long-term exposure of Mytilus galloprovincialis to diclofenac, Ibuprofen and Ketoprofen: Insights into bioavailability, biomarkers and transcriptomic changes. *Chemosphere.* 198:238-248.

Munari, M., Matozzo, V., Chemello, G., Riedl, V., Pastore, P., Badocco, D., Marin, M. G. 2019 Seawater acidification and emerging contaminants: A dangerous marriage for haemocytes of marine bivalves. *Environ Res.* 175:11-21.

Munari, M., Matozzo, V., Gagné, F., Chemello, G., Riedl, V., Finos, L., Pastore, P., Badocco, D., Marin, M. G. 2018 Does exposure to reduced pH and diclofenac induce oxidative stress in marine bivalves? A comparative study with the mussel Mytilus galloprovincialis and the clam Ruditapes philippinarum. *Environ Pollut.* 240:925-937.

Munari, M., Chemello, G., Finos, L., Ingrosso, G., Giani, M., Marin, M. G., 2016 Coping with seawater acidification and the emerging contaminant diclofenac at the larval stage: A tale from the clam Ruditapes philippinarum. *Chemosphere.* 160:293-302.

Nieto, E., Corada-Fernández, C., Hampel, M., Lara-Martín, P. A., Sánchez-Argüello, P., Blasco, J. 2017 Effects of exposure to pharmaceuticals (diclofenac and carbamazepine) spiked sediments in the midge, Chironomus riparius (Diptera, Chironomidae). *Sci Total Environ.* 31;609:715-723.

Önlü, S., Saçan, M. T. 2018 Toxicity of contaminants of emerging concern to Dugesia japonica: QSTR modeling and toxicity relationship with Daphnia magna J Hazard Mater. 351:20-28. Rand-Weaver M. 2013 The read-across Hypothesis and environmental risk Assessment of pharmaceuticals. *Environ. Sci. Technol.* 47:11384–11395.

Önlü, S., Saçan, M. T. 2017 An in silico algal toxicity model with a wide applicability potential for industrial chemicals and pharmaceuticals *Environ Toxicol Chem.* 36:1012-1019.

Önlü, S., Saçan, M. T. 2017 An in silico approach to cytotoxicity of pharmaceuticals and personal care products on the rainbow trout liver cell line RTL-W1. *Environ Toxicol Chem.* 36:1162-1169.

Osickova, J., Skochova, H., Ondracek, K., Kral, J., Damkova, V., Peckova, L., Pohanka, M., Vitula, F., Bandouchova, H., Pikula, J. 2012 Risk of single and combined exposure of birds to non-steroidal anti-inflammatory drugs and lead. *Neuro Endocrinol Lett* 33 Suppl 3:145-50.

Praskova, E., Voslarova, E., Siroka, Z., Plhalova, L., Macova, S., Marsalek, P., Pistekova, V., Svobodova, Z. 2011 Assessment of diclofenac LC50 reference values in juvenile and embryonic stages of the zebrafish (Danio rerio) *Polish Journal of Veterinary Sciences.* 14:545–549.

Praskova, E., Plhalova, L., Chromcova, L., Stepanova, S., Bedanova, I., Blahova, J., Hostovsky, M., Skoric, M., Maršálek, P., Voslarova, E., Svobodova, Z. 2014 Effects of subchronic exposure of diclofenac on growth, histopathological changes, and oxidative stress in zebrafish (Danio rerio). *Scientific World Journal* 645737.

Raisuddin, S., Kwok, K. W., Leung, K. M., Schlenk, D., Lee, J. S. 2007 The copepod Tigriopus: a promising marine model organism for ecotoxicology and environmental genomics. *Aquat Toxicol.* 83:161-73.

Ribas, J. L. C., Sherry, J. P., Zampronio, A. R., Silva de Assis H. C., Simmons D. B. D 2017 Inhibition of immune responses and related proteins in Rhamdia quelen exposed to diclofenac. *Environ Toxicol Chem.* 36:2092-2107.

Schmidt W., O'Rourke, K., Hernan, R., Quinn, B. 2011 Effects of the pharmaceuticals gemfibrozil and diclofenac on the marine mussel (Mytilus spp.) and their comparison with standardized toxicity tests. *Mar Pollut Bull.* 62:1389-95.

Schmidt, W., Rainville, L. C., McEneff, G., Sheehan, D., Quinn, B. 2014 A proteomic evaluation of the effects of the pharmaceuticals diclofenac and gemfibrozil on marine mussels (Mytilus spp.): evidence for chronic sublethal effects on stress-response proteins. *Drug Test Anal.* 26:210-9.

Schwaiger, J., Ferling, H., Mallow, U., Wintermayr, H., Negele, R. D. 2004 Toxic effects of the non-steroidal anti-inflammatory drug diclofenac. Part I: histopathological alterations and bioaccumulation in rainbow trout. *Aquat Toxicol.* 68:141-50.

Stringer, T. J, Glover, C. N., Keesing, V., Northcott, G. L., Gaw, S., Tremblay, L. A. 2014 Development of acute and chronic sediment bioassays with the harpacticoid copepod Quinquelaophonte sp. *Ecotoxicol Environ Saf.* 99:82-91.

Tang, J. Y. M., Mccarty, S., Glenn, E., Neale, P. A., Warne, M. S. J., Escher, B. I., 2013 Mixture effects of organic micropollutants present in water: Towards the development of effect-based water quality trigger values for baseline toxicity. *Water Res.* 47:3300–3314.

Toropova, A. P., Toropov A.A., Benfenati E., Gini G., Leszczynska D., Leszczynski J. Coral: 2012 Models of toxicity of binary mixtures. *Chemom. Intell. Lab. Syst.* 119:39–43.

Ukić Š, Sigurnjak M, Cvetnić M, Markić M, Stankov MN, Rogošić M, Rasulev B, Lončarić Božić A, Kušić H, Bolanča T. 2019 Toxicity of pharmaceuticals in binary mixtures: Assessment by additive and non-additive toxicity models. *Ecotoxicol Environ Saf.* 185:109696.

Van den Brandhof EJ, Montforts M. 2010 Fish embryo toxicity of carbamazepine, diclofenac and metoprolol. *Ecotoxicology and Environmental Safety.* 73:1862–1866.

Wang L, Peng Y, Nie X, Pan B, Ku P, Bao S 2016 Gene response of CYP360A, CYP314, and GST and whole-organism changes in Daphnia magna exposed to ibuprofen. *Comp Biochem Physiol C Toxicol Pharmacol.* 179:49-56.

Wang T., Wang D., Lin Z., An Q., Yin C., Huang O. 2016 Prediction of mixture toxicity from the hormesis of a single chemical: A case study of combinations of antibiotics and quorum-sensing inhibitors with gram-negative bacteria. *Chemosphere.* 150:159–167.

Wang J, He B, Yan D, Hu X 2017 Implementing ecopharmacovigilance (EPV) from a pharmacy perspective: A focus on non-steroidal anti-inflammatory drugs. *Sci Total Environ.* 603-604:772-784.

Wang J, Zhao SQ, Zhang MY, He BS 2018 Targeted eco-pharmacovigilance for ketoprofen in the environment: Need, strategy and challenge. *Chemosphere.* 194:450-462.

Yao Z., Lin Z., Wang T., Tian D., Zou X., Gao Y. 2013 Using molecular docking-based binding energy to predict toxicity of binary mixture with different binding sites. *Chemosphere.* 92:1169–1176.

Zou X., Lin Z., Deng Z., Yin D., Zhang Y. 2012 The joint effects of sulfonamides and their potentiator on photobacterium phosphoreum: Differences between the acute and chronic mixture toxicity mechanisms. *Chemosphere.* 86:30–35.

EDITOR'S CONTACT INFORMATION

Eugenia Yiannakopoulou
Academic Teacher
Department of Biomedical Sciences
Faculty of Health and Caring Professions,
University of West Attica, Athens Greece
Email: nyiannak@teiath.gr, nyiannak@uniwa.gr

INDEX

#

(2, 6-dichloranilino) phenylacetic acid, 38, 77, 90

A

ABA, 3, 22, 118
acid, 4, 6, 23, 24, 37, 38, 50, 65, 67, 70, 77, 82, 89, 90, 114, 118, 160
acidic, 52, 66
acute exposure, 60, 135, 152, 153, 156
adsorption, 52, 54, 79
advanced oxidation processes, 58, 74, 80, 130, 144
adverse effects, xi, 1, 3, 9, 10, 12, 17, 21, 39, 53, 108, 135, 149, 151
adverse event, 127, 129
ankylosing spondylitis, xiii, 49
antibiotic, 3, 19, 54
anti-inflammatory drugs, 22, 58, 74, 77, 121, 124
antioxidant enzymes, 129, 133, 134, 136, 156
antipyretic, xiii, 49
AOP, xiv, 74, 80, 84

aquatic life, 12
aquatic organisms, ix, xiii, xiv, 50, 52, 61, 105, 128, 133, 134, 152
Asia, 33, 34, 41, 46, 77
assessment, 2, 17, 22, 24, 62, 64, 68, 108, 132, 141, 150, 151, 162
avermectins, 10, 11, 22, 24
avian, 42, 47

B

bioaccumulation, 52, 69, 168
bioassays, 119, 141, 150, 153, 154, 159, 161, 162, 168
biodegradation, 10, 54, 58, 63, 122
biomarkers, 137, 145, 166
biomass, 133
bioremediation, xi, 2, 18
biotechnology, 110
biotic, 56, 57
birds, 33, 34, 35, 37, 40, 41, 42, 44, 46, 77, 112, 145, 167
blood, 38, 59, 64, 136, 142
breeding, xii, 11, 30, 40, 43, 45, 111
by-products, 89, 90, 92, 93, 134

Index

C

cabbage, 89
Cabinet, 26
cadmium, 144, 165
carbamazepine, 63, 108, 118, 119, 122, 146, 147, 166, 168
carbon, 52, 55, 57, 58, 63, 80, 82, 83, 86
carbon dioxide, 80, 82, 86
case study, 141, 162, 169
catalyst, 81, 82, 84, 87, 89
cattle, xv, 11, 22, 23, 24, 25, 26, 39, 46, 106
chemical, 6, 7, 13, 16, 17, 19, 21, 31, 38, 50, 51, 52, 59, 78, 79, 81, 107, 109, 113, 117, 139, 153, 155, 157, 158, 169
chemical characteristics, 52
chemical oxidation processes, 109
chemical properties, 108, 113, 159
chemicals, x, 1, 4, 13, 15, 19, 128, 131, 139, 150, 152, 157, 158
China, 39, 107, 125
chronic exposure, 60, 77, 129, 133, 137, 150, 153, 154, 155, 157, 159, 163
circadian rhythm, 136
classes, 35, 113
climate, xiv, 73, 75, 92
clinical implications, 106
clinical trials, 17, 112
clofibric acid, 4, 6
cocaine, 4, 6
computational approaches, 159
conduction, 85, 87, 88
conjugation, 115, 120
conservation, 39, 40, 43, 44, 45
consumption, xiii, 14, 50, 54, 69, 78, 79, 110
contaminant, 109, 117, 166
contaminated water, 110, 133
contamination, 37, 38, 67, 77
correlation, 59, 164
cost, 9, 79, 113, 153
crops, xv, 106, 114, 116, 148
curriculum, xv, 106, 117

D

DCF, xiv, 74, 77, 78, 79, 80, 84, 85, 89, 90, 91, 92, 93, 130
detoxification, 99, 115, 119, 156, 165
diclofenac, vii, viii, ix, x, xii, xiv, 4, 6, 22, 25, 29, 30, 32, 35, 36, 37, 38, 39, 40, 41, 42, 44, 45, 46, 47, 48, 49, 50, 51, 52, 53, 54, 56, 57, 58, 59, 60, 61, 63, 64, 65, 66, 67, 68, 70, 73, 74, 77, 94, 95, 96, 98, 99, 100, 101, 102, 105, 106, 108, 109, 110, 111, 113, 114, 115, 116, 117, 118, 119, 120, 121, 122, 123, 124, 127, 129, 130, 131, 132, 133, 134, 135, 136, 137, 138, 139, 140, 141, 142, 143, 144, 145, 146, 147, 148, 149, 150, 151, 152, 154, 155, 157, 158, 160, 161, 162, 163, 165, 166, 167, 168

E

eco- pharmacovigilance, 107
ecology, 3, 4, 7, 14, 20, 21, 31, 59, 65
ecopharmacology, xi, 4, 5, 7, 25, 31, 47
ecosystem, xii, 4, 7, 30, 31, 57, 128, 139, 154
ecotoxicological, 61, 115, 122, 145
ecotoxicology, 7, 31, 64, 67, 94, 95, 100, 141, 146, 147, 162, 165, 167, 169
effluent, 19, 24, 54, 78, 79
effluents, 19, 53, 63, 107, 127, 129
endangered, 34, 46, 48, 53, 122, 124
endocrine, xiv, 63, 73, 76, 155
energy, 75, 76, 81, 82, 84, 86, 88, 93
engineering, 86, 88
environment, ix, x, xii, xiv, 1, 3, 4, 6, 7, 8, 9, 11, 12, 13, 14, 15, 16, 17, 19, 20, 21, 22, 24, 27, 30, 31, 32, 44, 46, 52, 53, 56,

57, 60, 62, 63, 64, 65, 67, 68, 69, 70, 76, 80, 89, 105, 107, 108, 109, 112, 117, 118, 123, 125, 129, 130, 149, 151, 160, 169
environmental assessments, 23, 112
environmental conditions, 150, 160
environmental effects, 8, 11, 31, 59, 118, 153
environmental factors, 157
environmental impact, xi, xv, 2, 5, 8, 11, 20, 66, 106, 115, 150, 152, 157, 159
environmental levels, 50
environmental pharmacology, x, xv, 7, 26, 30, 106, 117, 129, 149, 151, 156, 157
environmental pharmacology of mixtures, 151
environmental risk, ix, xiv, 17, 62, 63, 64, 105, 107, 108, 109, 110, 111, 112, 117, 128, 131, 132, 137, 140, 150, 151, 153, 166
environmental toxicity, ix, xiii, xv, 42, 46, 50, 106, 113, 120, 128, 131, 134, 137, 139, 158, 160, 163
environmental toxicity of mixtures of pharmaceuticals, 159
enzymes, 15, 19, 129, 133, 134, 136, 138, 155, 163, 165
epidemiology, 14
estrogen, 24, 120, 121, 164
ethinyl estradio, 4, 6
European Commission, 56, 64
European Union, xi, 2, 3, 16, 17, 18, 27, 78, 129

F

fate, 24, 25, 50, 52, 53, 55, 65, 66, 67, 70, 89, 94, 96, 98, 99, 101, 102, 103, 107, 124, 147
food, x, xiii, xv, 4, 12, 16, 32, 36, 40, 44, 45, 50, 106, 114, 154

Food and Drug Administration, 22
food chain, xiii, 4, 16, 32, 40, 50, 154
formation, 37, 85, 86, 89, 90, 91, 93, 114, 119
free radicals, 137, 138
freshwater, xv, 7, 53, 57, 65, 66, 75, 76, 92, 106, 110, 117, 142, 162, 165
fungi, 19, 110
fungus, 110, 122

H

harmful effects, xi, xv, 1, 4, 106, 117
health, x, xiii, xv, 5, 12, 14, 18, 21, 26, 33, 39, 49, 63, 66, 76, 106, 107, 116, 117, 122, 123, 124, 140
homeostasis, 128, 131, 135, 138
hormones, 3, 6, 10, 17, 70
human, ix, xi, xiii, xv, 2, 4, 8, 9, 12, 14, 15, 16, 17, 20, 21, 22, 29, 31, 32, 39, 40, 50, 53, 54, 60, 64, 75, 76, 106, 110, 113, 115, 116, 118, 123, 125, 127, 129, 145, 146, 156, 157
human exposure, ix, xv, 12, 106, 113, 116
human health, ix, xv, 40, 106, 110, 113, 115, 116, 117, 123, 125
hydrogen, 81, 99, 138
hydrogen peroxide, 81, 138
hypoxia, 136, 143

I

ibuprofen, 10, 22, 39, 66, 67, 68, 111, 142, 146, 169
iclofenac, ix, xv, 106, 111, 133, 136, 156
ideal, 20
identification, 65, 150, 152
idiosyncratic, 43, 154
illumination, 84, 88
immune response, 167
improvements, 14, 21

in silico approaches, 151, 160
in silico tools, 113
in vitro, 159
in vivo, 159
incidence, 38
India, ix, xii, xv, 1, 9, 29, 30, 33, 34, 35, 36, 37, 38, 39, 40, 41, 43, 45, 46, 47, 48, 106, 107, 110, 116, 119, 124, 150, 151, 162
individuals, 5, 21
induction, 128, 131, 138, 139
industrialization, xiv, 73, 75, 92
industry, 15, 20, 26, 40
inflammation, xiii, 49, 51, 77, 111
ingestion, 50, 55, 77, 110
ingredients, xiv, 3, 5, 12, 21, 58, 62, 74
inhibition, 37, 61, 115, 136, 156
invertebrates, 10, 110, 155
irrigation, 107, 116, 123, 125
issues, x, xiv, 74, 128, 137, 150, 151, 152, 155

M

mass, 69, 70, 78, 114
mass spectrometry, 70
materials, 45, 84, 86
measurement, 52, 137, 140
measurement of oxidative stress, 137, 140
medical, x, xii, 3, 9, 21, 30, 32
medical science, xii, 30
medicine, xi, xii, xv, 10, 14, 16, 20, 29, 35, 49, 51, 106, 117
metabolic pathways, 114, 128, 139
metabolism, 13, 15, 42, 107, 114, 130, 133, 154, 156
metabolites, ix, xi, xiii, xv, 2, 4, 15, 21, 24, 32, 50, 62, 106, 109, 112, 113, 114, 123, 130, 133, 145
metabolized, 4, 15, 32, 41, 112, 130

methodological issues, 128, 137, 150, 151, 152
methodology, x, 46, 120, 153, 163
milbemycins, 10
mineralization, 58, 89, 91, 92
models, 42, 113, 119, 131, 168
molecules, xiii, 13, 19, 50, 59, 62, 85
mortality, 34, 35, 45, 48, 90
mortality rate, 34, 90
multiple agents, 151
mussels, 128, 133, 134, 141, 155, 158, 162, 168

N

Na^+, 51
Na_2SO_4, 58
necrosis, 36, 38, 157
negative consequences, 117
negative effects, 23
Nepal, xii, 30, 37, 38, 41, 43, 44, 45
nephrosis, 42
neutral, 91, 158
Nile, 163
nitrogen, 132
NMR, 101
non steroidal anti-inflammatory, 127, 129, 137, 150, 151
non-steroidal anti-inflammatory drugs, 120, 125, 167, 169
NSAIDs, xii, 30, 36, 37, 39, 46, 77, 111, 127, 129
nursing, 20
nursing home, 20
nutrient, 24, 38
nutrients, 110

P

pain, 3, 6, 10, 51

Pakistan, ix, xii, xv, 25, 30, 33, 35, 36, 38, 41, 43, 47, 67, 106, 110, 116, 122, 150, 151
pH, 52, 63, 82, 89, 91, 135, 144, 158, 166
pharmaceutical, x, xiv, 1, 9, 12, 13, 15, 18, 20, 24, 26, 40, 50, 53, 58, 62, 65, 66, 67, 70, 73, 77, 92, 107, 108, 118, 121, 122, 123, 125, 126, 127, 129, 140, 146, 154, 158, 161, 164
pharmaceuticals, ix, x, xiv, 1, 3, 7, 9, 12, 13, 16, 17, 20, 21, 22, 24, 31, 44, 51, 52, 53, 55, 64, 65, 66, 67, 68, 69, 70, 76, 77, 78, 105, 107, 109, 110, 112, 113, 116, 117, 118, 119, 120, 123, 124, 125, 126, 130, 132, 133, 140, 141, 143, 146, 149, 151, 153, 154, 158,159, 160, 161, 163, 166, 167, 168
Pharmaceuticals and Personal Care Products (PPCPs), 5, 6, 7, 15, 23, 31, 42, 47, 65, 97, 98, 125
pharmaceutics, 7, 18, 31
pharmacoenvironmentology, xii, 2, 26, 30, 47
pharmacokinetics, 25, 47, 52, 107
pharmacological agents, 5, 8
pharmacology, x, xv, 4, 7, 26, 30, 31, 106, 107, 117, 128, 129, 149, 151, 156, 157
pharmacotherapy, 4, 8, 32
pharmacovigilance, vii, x, xi, 1, 2, 5, 7, 8, 14, 21, 25, 26, 27, 29, 30, 31, 32, 47, 108, 111, 120, 125, 160, 169
phenylbutazone, 39
phosphorus, 11
photocatalysis, xiv, 74, 81, 83, 84, 86, 89, 92, 95, 96, 98, 99, 100
photodegradation, 63, 91, 93
photolysis, 58, 89, 109, 120, 130, 134, 141
photosynthesis, 115, 123, 132
photo-transformation, 61
physicochemical properties, 159
physiology, 77, 128, 139, 145, 154, 155
phytoremediation, 18

plants, ix, xiii, xv, 3, 6, 9, 19, 50, 53, 56, 66, 67, 68, 70, 74, 78, 89, 97, 98, 101, 102, 106, 109, 111, 112, 113, 114, 115, 119, 120, 121, 123, 124, 126, 128, 130, 132, 133, 143, 145, 147, 153, 154
policy, x, xiii, 18, 50, 62
pollutant, 52, 53, 56, 62, 79, 82, 89, 130, 132
pollutants, 7, 18, 31, 79, 84, 88, 108, 140, 144, 154, 161
pollution, xiii, xiv, 6, 14, 50, 73, 75, 76, 92, 145
population, ix, xi, xii, xiv, xv, 2, 16, 17, 24, 25, 30, 32, 33, 35, 40, 44, 45, 46, 47, 48, 61, 67, 73, 77, 106, 110, 116, 119, 120, 122, 150, 151, 162, 164
population growth, xiv, 73
potassium, 39, 51, 52, 58
predators, 4, 32, 39, 57
Prediction of Environmental Risk, 112
prevention, 2, 14, 108, 128, 131, 139
proliferation, 77, 111, 158
protection, 14, 64, 138
proteins, 167, 168
proximal convoluted tubules, 36, 38

R

radicals, 58, 85, 86, 90, 130, 131, 137
reactions, 2, 8, 32, 85, 114
reactive oxygen, 132
residues, 9, 11, 12, 14, 20, 21, 23, 25, 26, 37, 38, 46, 47, 48, 52, 65, 67, 118, 119, 122, 123, 124, 162
response, 8, 38, 112, 120, 128, 131, 135, 140, 142, 147, 148, 162, 168, 169
risks, ix, xi, xii, xiii, xiv, 2, 10, 11, 12, 17, 22, 25, 30, 33, 39, 40, 42, 50, 60, 62, 63, 64, 66, 74, 77, 80, 92, 99, 105, 107, 109, 110, 112, 116, 117, 120, 122, 123, 125, 132, 140, 143, 150, 151, 160, 164, 167

roots, xv, 106, 114, 133
routes, xi, 1, 109
Royal Society, 36, 44
rutile, 86

S

safety, xi, xvi, 2, 12, 29, 40, 41, 42, 106, 117
scavengers, xii, xv, 30, 44, 106, 110, 116, 119
sediment, xiii, 50, 55, 57, 66, 168
sediments, 52, 65, 68, 69, 111, 166
semiconductor, 81, 82, 84, 88, 89
semiconductors, 81, 82, 86, 87
sensitization, 87, 88, 89, 93
sewage, 3, 6, 12, 21, 24, 65, 107
sexual development, 121, 164
silico tools, 113
sludge, 52, 54, 63, 66, 107, 125, 130
sodium, 4, 6, 39, 50, 51, 52, 142
solution, xiv, 17, 19, 40, 74, 89, 90, 91, 92, 93
South Asia, xii, 30, 32, 33, 36, 67
species, ix, xv, 19, 25, 26, 33, 34, 35, 36, 37, 39, 41, 42, 43, 47, 48, 58, 60, 61, 90, 106, 107, 110, 111, 112, 115, 116, 118, 121, 122, 129, 132, 139, 140, 150, 152, 153, 154, 157, 160, 161, 165
stakeholders, 60, 61
states, ix, xv, 106, 111
stress, 115, 128, 131, 132, 133, 134, 135, 136, 137, 138, 139, 140, 142, 144, 145, 147, 163, 165, 168
stress response, 115, 128, 131, 134, 135, 138, 140, 147
stressors, 128, 131, 134, 136
structure, 13, 16, 70, 113, 150, 159, 160, 161
sulfate, 19, 58, 114
sulfonamides, 169

Sun, 80, 81, 97, 126
survival, 12, 25, 26, 42, 155
Switzerland, 79, 99
synergistic effect, 91, 93

T

target, xiii, 50, 53, 61, 107, 112, 116, 117, 128, 131, 132, 136, 137, 138, 139, 150, 153, 155, 157, 160
Targeted ecopharmacovigilance, 160
teachers, x
techniques, xi, 2, 18, 54
technological advances, 3
technologies, 76, 80, 84, 109, 117, 125
technology, 16, 31, 81, 86, 143
temperature, 59, 134, 141, 158, 162
testing, 9, 16, 17, 37, 42, 46, 115, 120, 161, 163
toxic, x, xiv, 10, 20, 35, 36, 42, 65, 69, 74, 76, 77, 78, 82, 89, 90, 91, 92, 93, 118, 128, 129, 130, 131, 140, 152, 161, 165, 168
toxic effect, x, xiv, 20, 35, 42, 74, 77, 92, 93, 118, 128, 129, 131, 140, 152, 161
toxicity, ix, xiii, xv, 10, 11, 22, 39, 42, 46, 49, 50, 53, 58, 60, 61, 64, 67, 77, 78, 90, 91, 92, 93, 106, 113, 119, 120, 121, 128, 131, 134, 136, 137, 138, 139, 141, 142, 143, 146, 147, 150, 152, 153, 154, 156, 158, 160, 161, 162, 163, 164, 166, 168, 169

V

vultures extinction, 30

W

waste, 6, 7, 13, 19, 54, 67, 79, 127, 129

wastewater, xiii, xv, 9, 16, 19, 50, 53, 56, 57, 59, 64, 66, 68, 69, 70, 71, 76, 78, 83, 92, 106, 109, 111, 116, 117, 123, 124, 125, 130, 141, 144, 145, 146, 147
water, xiv, 3, 6, 9, 12, 13, 15, 24, 52, 54, 57, 58, 61, 62, 63, 69, 70, 73, 75, 76, 77, 79, 80, 82, 83, 84, 85, 89, 90, 92, 99, 108, 109, 110, 111, 113, 116, 119, 122, 126, 130, 143, 144, 152, 158, 168
wells, x, 113, 154

WHO, 7, 18, 20, 31
wide band gap, 93
wildlife, 34, 39, 44, 107, 154
wildlife conservation, 34
withdrawal, xii, 30, 41
World Health Organization, 2, 108
worldwide, ix, xiv, 54, 106, 109, 122, 127, 129, 152